So Your Pet Has Cancer... Now What?

So Your Pet Has Cancer... Now What?

An Integrative Veterinary Oncologist's Guide to Empower You Through This Journey

DR. ERIN BANNINK
DVM, DIPLOMATE ACVIM (ONCOLOGY)
Integrative Specialist | Metaphysical Teacher | Spiritual Guide

GOLDEN ACORN
PRESS

NAPLES, FL

Published in the United States by Golden Acorn Press, Naples, Florida, United States of America
www.goldenacornpress.com

ISBN: (print) 979-8-950207-04-4
ISBN: (ebook) 979-8-950207-05-1
Cataloging-in-Publication Data is on file with the Library of Congress.

Developmental Editing by Heather Davis Desrocher
Line Editing by Jennifer Doody
Proofreading by David Aretha
Cover and Interior Design by Jessica Angerstein

Printed in the United States of America

To my mom, who opened so many doors for me to be myself
and showed me there is more than one way to view the world.

To my dad, who taught me to be strong.

To my husband, who loves and supports me in ways that any
expression of gratitude would fall short of adequately honoring.

To my patients and clients,
who give me a reason to serve, love, learn and grow.

You are all the reason I am here.

Contents

PART IV THE SPIRIT

Foreword by

Dr. Kendra Pope, DVM, DACVIM (Oncology)

It is my great honor to write the foreword to *So Your Pet Has Cancer...Now What?* As a board-certified veterinary oncologist and one of the few integrative veterinary oncologists practicing in the United States alongside Dr. Erin Bannink, I know first-hand how rare and needed this book is.

For more than a decade, I have sat across from pet parents in the moments after a cancer diagnosis. I know the look in their eyes – the shock, the grief, the desperate question of *What do I do now*? In those moments, a treatment plan is rarely enough. What pet parents truly need is clarity, options and a road map for the whole journey, one that honors both the science of cancer care and the sacred bond they share with their animal. That is exactly what Erin has created in this book.

What makes this book so powerful is that Erin does not stop at treatment; instead, she begins where conventional resources end. With the steady hand of a clinician and the open heart of a healer, she guides the reader through the Three Cornerstones of Whole-Being Wellness – Body, Soul and Spirit – offering a framework I have not seen captured this completely anywhere else. She gives readers permission to grieve, tools to steady themselves, and a way to walk this journey with intention rather than fear.

What makes this book so valuable is that Erin understands something most cancer guides miss: The pet parent is not a bystander in this story. They are the most important variable in their pet's experience. Erin shows you how to step into that role with strength and grace, and in doing so, transform one of life's most painful chapters into one of the most meaningful. Few practitioners can move as fluently as Erin does between the science of medicine and the wisdom of the spirit, and it is precisely that rare combination that gives this book its depth.

This book belongs in the hands of every pet parent navigating a cancer diagnosis, every veterinarian who wants to better support their clients, and anyone who has ever loved an animal deeply enough to want to honor that bond fully. Erin has given us a true gift – a guide that meets people in their grief and walks them all the way home to peace. Turn the page. You are in good hands.

Dr. Kendra Pope, DVM, DACVIM (Oncology), cTCVMP
Founder & Medical Director, Prism Integrative Veterinary Health Founder, Prism Veterinary Research Institute

Preface

You Are the Sun in Your Pet's Universe

If your pet has been diagnosed with cancer, you may be worried, grieving or overwhelmed. Maybe you are fiercely motivated to explore every option to help them. Maybe you feel helpless. This is often the first area I address with my clients. There is always something you can do. Focusing on where you DO have power is very important now. This is why I wrote this book; because there is so much more than you may have been told. And you hold the key to it all.

Through the course of this book I am going to offer you a way through the brambles of worry, overwhelm, grief and stress that honors the bond you share with your pet. I will of course share what you need to know, including treatments, but I want to offer you so much more than that! This book is a way through the journey of your pet's cancer that focuses on the gift of life, the sacredness of your relationship, and the power of your Spirit.

This book speaks to the depth of power that lies within you. Maybe it's dormant. Maybe it's just a little jostled right now. Nonetheless, it is there and can be your guiding light. You just need to reach in and access it, and then choose to use it.

You are infinitely more powerful than you think you are. You are capable of so much. And there is a way to live life that brings you into a state of inner peace that will carry you through the challenges with strength, calm and clarity. Love is a powerful force. And I know you have a lot of that inside of you. That Love will be your greatest source of strength and power now. Love is the force that will carry you through this and provide the fortitude you need.

To your pet, you are the center of the universe: You are their Sun. Their life revolves around you. Pets do not understand that they have cancer like people do. They only know how they feel *now,* and they take their cues from you. As the Sun in their universe, you are the biggest part of their day-to-day experience. When their Sun shines brightly, their life is better.

What you do now and how you support yourself in navigating this journey matters a great deal not only to your quality of life, but to theirs too.

This book will equip you with tools to rewrite your experience in a way that will support you not only through the current journey, but long after this chapter with your pet is complete. It will help you transform your script of grief, anxiety and overwhelm into a story of hope, healing and learning. And in the end, regardless of how this chapter ultimately finds its conclusion, you will have a greater appreciation for the beauty of the powerful bond you share with your pet.

By choosing to take this precious being into your care, you have received the gifts of growth and love. In return, your pet will need your best self on this journey. So it is time to step fully into your power. Let me show you how.

A diagnosis is not the end of the story.
It is an invitation to discover strengths, wisdom and love you may never have known are already within you.

Introduction

The Choice

Learning that your pet has cancer is heartbreaking. Our animal companions have shared so much life with us. They have often shared important moments and accompanied us through major life events, transitions or even tragedies. They have been a source of comfort during difficult times, a steady source of nonjudgmental companionship and unconditional acceptance. I have many clients who tell me their dog or cat is their best friend or like their child. I understand. Our pets can be like our children in many ways. They are a member of our family, and they ask so little of us in return. That unconditional love can bring healing, one of the miracles of the human-animal bond.

I know it is hard to imagine journeying through the cancer diagnosis. The diagnosis of cancer itself often brings with it a storm of fears and emotions that is unique from other diseases. Just the thought itself can feel paralyzing. Almost all of my clients tell me their primary concern is that their pet has the best quality of life possible for whatever time they have left; that above all, they don't want them to suffer. The love we have for them can create an inner conflict between not wanting to lose them, not wanting them to suffer, and being afraid of making the wrong decisions.

When you receive a diagnosis of cancer in your pet, grief may hit. Even though you know they are still here and might even feel fine right now, you are grieving a future loss that hasn't happened yet. That is called anticipatory grief. It is very real and very normal. Hopefully, you have good support around you, but it isn't unusual to find that others may have a hard time understanding the depth of your sadness. They don't feel your bond with your pet. You may be feeling things that you think you shouldn't be feeling, or that others say you shouldn't be feeling.

It is important to be gentle with yourself during this time as you take the next delicate steps down this cancer care journey. You will need a way to rest your mind and quiet your racing thoughts. Maybe you will need to take more walks in nature. Seek out more time for rest. Talk with a trusted friend or therapist to help you sort through the complexities of all you are feeling. Maybe you will dive into information, setting yourself on a mission to find answers. Maybe, inspired by the information in this book, you will incorporate new modalities of healing you hadn't considered before.

No matter what you need as an individual, one thing is universally true: Within the pain, there is a seed of opportunity.

Even though it may seem difficult to access right now, if I have learned anything in life, it is that what we choose to do with our experiences determines whether we merely survive or whether we grow through the experience. There are gifts hidden in every challenge. It is up to us to decide what to do with the situations in our life. Are you going to lose yourself in this? Or will you choose to lean in and find the opportunities to grow?

I am not here to belittle life's challenges or to suggest you ignore the pain. I also won't suggest that you be grateful for difficult experiences. That would not be kind, compassionate or helpful. You need to go through your emotions in a healthy way. And there is a way to shift the focus of this journey from the difficulties to the opportunities – from feelings of helplessness and overwhelm to the places you do have control, where you can make a positive impact.

Let's start by asking: How can we make this cancer journey the best one possible? You might say, "That's a nice idea. But how? This is overwhelming and painful and I don't want this to be happening." What if you could turn this challenge into an opportunity for growth and healing? Through challenges, we are able to know ourselves better. We are able to discover the depths of our strengths, the places within us that need attention, and the true extent of our current capacities.

It would be nice if we could grow without going through challenges. But when we are comfortable, we tend to just cruise on autopilot. Challenges are the way we really see what we are made of, how we stretch ourselves, and become more than we are today. My most painful and difficult experiences were also the strongest motivators for my own growth, and they ultimately resulted in the most positive personal transformations. They motivated me to look for better answers to my suffering and the questions I had about life, healing and success. Those experiences guided me to the threshold of doors I would never have known existed, had it not been for the hardships that drove me to seek a better way and explore new territories of growth and healing.

I also have a very real appreciation for the blocks and resistances that come up while in the midst of intense emotions and challenging life events. I know that it can often be extremely difficult to pick yourself up and find a clear path forward on your own when in the cloud of overwhelm. This book will serve as a guiding light for you as you navigate your journey, and remind you that you are not alone. It will provide you with a way to focus your energies and remember that you are an amazing and powerful person, even if you don't believe that right now. This book won't solve all your problems. It won't reveal some new "magic bullet" treatment or supplement or diet to cure cancer. Why? Because the magic bullet is You.

This book will help you focus on the things YOU can do. It will walk you through a process that will support you, and will take you deeper than the face value of things. It may invite you to think differently than you do now. It may challenge you to release limiting beliefs about yourself. The focus on Whole-Being Wellness and caring for your Soul and Spirit will help you redefine success as it relates to the experience of the cancer journey, and maybe even to life.

If you put what is outlined here into practice, this book will empower you to create the best possible experience for yourself and your pet as you navigate a cancer diagnosis. My hope is that you will one day be able to look back on this experience, and even if you say, "That was painful, and I never want to go through that again," you will also say, "...and I have peace around it because I did the best I could possibly do for both of us." And, "I learned so much about myself and am grateful for the ways I have grown. I am a better version of myself now than I was before."

Why do I want that? Because you are going through this journey either way. You have an opportunity to choose to grow through the journey and become the lasting legacy of your pet's life. There is no better way to honor them than to learn everything your relationship with them has to teach you. That is how they truly live forever – through you and the positive things you do in the world. Those ripple out, leaving a wake of positive change that lives even beyond your life, and carries on in a legacy of love for future generations. And that will empower you to make the gift of the time you have with them all the better.

How to Use This Book

This book is designed to walk you through a process of expansion in the way you approach this journey with your pet. It invites you to go beyond the mind and the physicality of the cancer diagnosis. There are many books about treatment protocols, supplements and diet. This book is not about giving you a treatment protocol. It is about giving you a protocol to LIVE better through this journey, make decisions that honor both the mind and heart, and develop a deeper understanding of your power.

Science keeps us grounded and helps us make decisions, but it does not speak to the whole of who we are in the journey of healing. Rather, it speaks to the mind. There will be science in this book, for grounding and reference, but this journey with your pet is about much more than science, medicine and cancer. It is about love. It is about the power of the human-animal bond. Love arises from your Spirit and speaks to your heart, not your mind. Love fuels the passion to help and moves you to look for better answers. Love is what transforms us and heals us, Body, Soul and Spirit. The echoes of that love are what stay with you forever.

This book is really about the Soul and Spirit of caring for your pet after their cancer diagnosis. It is about connecting with the DEEPER layers of healing that are the reason the human-animal bond is such a powerful experience.

We will start first with the physical body and the practicalities of the decisions you face at the start of the pet cancer journey. Part I of this book is based on the most commonly asked questions I receive from clients, common concerns, and the common places where I see people struggle the most at this stage. If you are already well past this or reading this book to support your healthy pet, you may choose to skip this section of the book.

At the end of each chapter is a summary or reflection activity to help you connect with and remember the main points of the chapter. These "Check-In" pages are designed to support you in creating a Whole-Being Wellness lifestyle. They are also a powerful place for you to revisit periodically, to help you reconnect with the concepts as your journey progresses.

In addition, at the end of each of the four parts of this book is a "Diving Deeper" chapter. This chapter invites you to think bigger. If this isn't your cup of tea or it feels like too much right now, just skip these chapters. You can always come back to them later. These, however, are my favorite things to talk about, and I have found them the most interesting part of my personal journey to gaining a better understanding of life and myself.

Ultimately, just reading this book itself won't change anything. What you choose to change, and to DO every day with what you learn, is what creates the change to a new way of being. This book is a road map, and you don't simply read a road map. You use it to chart the path to a destination that you then physically follow – not just in your mind, intention and thoughts, but through real-life action. By the end of this book, you will have a road map to the Three Cornerstones of Whole-Being Wellness, which you can use in your everyday life to support you and your pet through this journey.

Three Cornerstones of Wellness

Modern medicine has come a long way in addressing many diseases and serious injuries of the physical body. Psychology provides methods to work with thoughts and emotions, helping you learn to process them in a healthy way. The more subtle and spiritual aspects of your wellness are very often overlooked in the modern era, but they are no less important. These aspects play an integral role in the health, balance and wellness of the physical body, mind and emotions. In order to achieve Whole-Being Wellness, there must be balance in all three cornerstones of wellness: Body, Soul and Spirit. If any one of these is neglected, balance is not truly achieved.

You very likely have done significant personal work yourself already. Many people who are interested in health and healing have explored a wide variety of healing modalities. If you are like many of my clients, you may fall into one of these categories:

1. "I know there must be something more to life, but I've not been able to connect with a deep well of internal meaning and purpose. I have found that in my relationship with my pet. Now my pet is sick and I can't imagine living without him."
2. "I struggle with self-worth and find it difficult to take care of myself in the ways I know would help me. But I will do anything for my pet."

3. "I have a pretty good self-care routine and a spiritual practice that I engage with at least occasionally, but this cancer diagnosis has really sent me into a tailspin and I don't know where to go from here."
4. "I've tried 'everything' and still feel like there is something missing in my life. I am very motivated and am good at getting things done. I am mission-driven and am not afraid to put the work in to achieve something better for myself and those I love. But I need a clear direction."

Where do you see yourself in this journey? Here is another way to frame the above experiences. Which one do you resonate with most strongly?

1. **Heart-Seeker:** You are searching for deeper meaning and connection, often finding it through your pet. *Yearning is awakening. You sense there's "something more" but are unsure how to access it. You find deep meaning through your pet. You are learning to use that love to open a door to greater purpose.*
2. **Devoted Giver:** You struggle with self-worth but pour love and care into your pet. *You often neglect yourself but rise fiercely in devotion for those you love. Your love burns brightly for others – now you are learning to turn that love inward.*
3. **Shaken Soul:** You had a foundation but feel lost after the cancer diagnosis. *You have some spiritual grounding but that has been destabilized by the cancer diagnosis. Your compass has been shaken, and you are seeking grounding and*

guidance. Once rooted, you are now awakening to deeper layers of strength.

4. **Purpose-Driven Pathfinder:** You are a high-achieving, mission-oriented individual craving deeper alignment and clarity. *You are motivated and capable, but seeking a soul-aligned map for what's next. You have done the work and seek true alignment with a higher purpose. Mission-driven and ready, you seek to walk in full Soul alignment.*

No matter where you fall on this spectrum, there is hope. And there is a path you can walk, as far as you choose, into greater well-being for you and your pet in the face of this cancer diagnosis.

In my experience, the most common missing piece in achieving Whole-Being Wellness is the deeper healing that gets to the level of the Soul and Spirit. This is especially true if you are feeling a lack of zest for life, a lack of hope, or that life is lacking meaning or purpose. This is also a common thread that weaves its way into feelings of depression, anxiety and apathy. Building a wellness lifestyle that begins to bridge the spiritual and physical parts of life brings Soul healing, which will benefit you both.

This is a healing journey you and your pet can walk together. The human-animal bond has a special kind of beauty. The reason it feels "Soul deep" is that it connects with one of our basic human needs: Love. That love can be the fuel that re-ignites our will to make positive adjustments. It can help us heal the places inside of us where we reject love, or where we refuse to love ourselves.

There is a powerful synergy within the human-animal bond. Animals remind us that we are worthy of love. In turn, as we connect with that flow of love and give it in return, we are uplifted. We shine more brightly. As the Sun in your pet's universe, when you shine brightly, their life is better. You now have the opportunity to use the gift of their love, and the bond you share, to help you step into a new version of life in which you are empowered and connected more deeply to a larger meaning and purpose in life.

Maybe you have struggled with your weight and your pet is overweight as well. I have had clients who went on a diet with their dog or cat and they both achieved better health. I have had many clients change the way they eat after learning about new ways to think about the impact of food, food processing and chemical exposure. I have clients who exercise more because they are exercising with and for their pet. I have also had clients who have chosen to work with me through my Divine Power-House Healing Center. By choosing to achieve their own inner healing to support them through the pet cancer journey, they have experienced deep shifts in their own well-being. Many of these clients truly believe their pet brought them to me so THEY could heal through the experience. I believe that many pets are not "normal" pets. The power of the bond they share with their humans is more than a simple animal companion. I have seen pets that are helping their humans in ways their humans don't understand.

You now have the opportunity to turn the challenge of a cancer diagnosis into inspiration to heal at an even deeper level, one that honors the nature of the human-animal bond. Just as you are evolving through your life experiences, animals that live as close members of your family evolve through your love, care and nurturing as individual beings who bring great meaning to your life. You are helping them too, far beyond tending to their physical needs.

Beliefs

Information doesn't change people's belief systems; *experience* does.

I am going to share a perspective with you that I hope will help you, fully realizing that until you have a new experience, the words in this book will not change what you believe to be true. Until you have a concept in your mind, you can't think about yourself or the world around you in a new way. It isn't available to you. That is one of the reasons exposing ourselves to new ways of thinking is so important to our continued growth and forward movement. It opens the door to new experiences.

My hope is that you will take what I am sharing here, mull it over, and then try it out. Apply it to your life. Test it. If you do that, you will have new experiences that will help you shift. When you are ready for more, there are steps you can take to reach new levels in life, and practices that help you navigate challenging times with more ease and grace. We will get to that later, in Part IV.

PART 1

PREPARING FOR THE JOURNEY

A Balanced Perspective

Cancer treatment is a multifaceted challenge. At the heart of this challenge lies the human component. The emotional and psychological trauma that often accompanies a cancer diagnosis can greatly affect the development of an optimal treatment plan for an individual patient or family. Family circumstances, belief systems, and goals for the life of a family pet must be central to a compassionate approach to patient care.

The Power of Your Bond

The influence of the human-animal bond is widely acknowledged. Just look at the number of emotional support animals and the studies showing the health benefits of animal companions. The phenomenon of the human-animal bond affects us deeply. A cancer diagnosis in a treasured animal companion is devastating news. Especially with the increasing stressors of everyday life, many people become overwhelmed. This impact of pet cancer is far-reaching, with an estimated 12 million dogs and cats diagnosed with cancer each year in the United States alone.[1]

It is important to understand we are all connected. While pets affect us, we also affect them. Healing is also multifactorial. Sometimes we heal *from* the events in our life. Sometimes we heal *through* them. As much as we want to avoid it, pain is a part of life, just as pleasure is a part of life. These are just opposite poles on the spectrum of our human experience. As long as we are alive, painful things will happen. We may not have a choice about what happens or how, but we always do have a choice about what we do with the situations in which we find ourselves.

In my practice I have worked with thousands of pets and their humans. I have seen firsthand the different ways people can move through this cancer journey with a pet. Let me share two real-life stories that may help you choose how you want to move through this journey.

Jane loved her dog, Blaze. When Blaze was diagnosed with cancer, Jane was determined to do everything she could. It was hard for her to imagine living without her best friend by her side. Although she decided on a treatment plan, she constantly questioned it, worried she had made the wrong decision. She continued to scour the internet for the newest miracle, and she questioned Blaze's doctors at every visit, rehashing the options and bringing in printouts of things she had researched that promised results.

Jane just couldn't accept that there wasn't something more that could be done. Her search, and the feeling she was missing something that would provide the guaranteed cure she so desperately wanted, occupied most of her waking moments. She cried daily. She didn't sleep. And when she did, it was fitful. She was constantly watching Blaze, worried something terrible was about to happen. Every cough or sneeze sent her into a panic.

Months went by like this. Her quality of life declined. She stopped doing things she enjoyed because she was afraid to leave Blaze alone. She spent her limited income on his treatments, and neglected her own health. She was exhausted, and every day felt overwhelming. Blaze seemed to be getting more and more anxious, even though the oncologist confirmed Blaze's cancer was in remission. Jane was just waiting for things to get worse, regularly dreading the day she would need to say goodbye to her best friend. And every day Blaze was there, wagging his tail, wondering why Jane was so sad.

Contrast Jane's story with Mary's: Mary loved her dog, Pepper. When Pepper was diagnosed with cancer, Mary was determined to do everything she could. She couldn't imagine living without her best friend by her side. She had taken Pepper into her care knowing that his companionship would last maybe a decade, being a large dog, and she was determined to make the most of the time they had. She carefully considered all the options, weighed them against her goals for Pepper's life and the current realities of her resources, and decided on a treatment plan. Mary knew there was no way to predict what would happen for Pepper. She knew in her heart that she was doing the best she could for him, and this gave her some peace around her choices. She decided the best way for her to move forward was to focus on the things she could control.

Mary prepared Pepper's meals with love, even when she couldn't feed him the fanciest food. She took intentional walks with him, allowing herself to focus on the gift of each moment: the beauty surrounding them, and the gratitude that she was given the opportunity to have such a wonderful dog. Mary stepped up her self-care and scheduled regular healing sessions for herself, because she knew this new stress might make things harder if she didn't take better care of herself too.

Mary still felt sad some days, and she gave herself permission to cry when she needed to just let that out. But she didn't dwell on the worry or the grief. She allowed herself to truly appreciate the special moments she and Pepper shared, and to let the love she experienced fill her up and sustain her through any worries.

She made a list of things Pepper loved to do, and decided to enjoy those adventures together. She focused on living and on giving them both the best quality of life.

Every day became an opportunity to learn and grow. Mary learned so much about wellness and how to support them both. She started taking better care of herself because she noticed that when she did she felt better, and it was important for her to be at her best – if not for her, then for Pepper. Mary discovered new levels of strength and capability. She knew Pepper had no idea he was sick, although the diagnosis of cancer was changing their routine. She did her best to live in the moment. And every day Pepper was there, wagging his tail and content, as Mary became more and more at peace and seemed more in the present moment; not only with Pepper, but with the people who came to visit them.

Sparked by her passion to help Pepper, Mary discovered things about herself she never would have known. Her relationships with the people in her life grew stronger, as she appreciated them in a new way. In her determination to make the best of the situation in front of them, she stepped onto a path that ended up connecting her to a bigger mission and purpose. Pepper's life, love and story lived on through Mary, forever making a difference in all the lives she touched.

You can see there are very different ways to move through this experience. Your presence and the way you focus your attention has the potential to shift the tone of the experience for both you and your pet. The choice is yours, and I am here to guide you through this process.

Since my residency days, it has always been a dream of mine to have a practice in which, while I am treating my veterinary patients, I also have services to support my pet parents through the cancer journey with modalities that work on our nonphysical aspects too – and now I can offer both (more on that later). So much human suffering can be alleviated, and so many opportunities for growth can be harnessed, when we embrace and give attention to all the dimensions of our experience.

It is also important to remember you are not alone. If you find you need and want support, there are resources at the end of this book for you to explore.

Healing begins the moment our attention shifts from fighting what we fear to nurturing what we love.

Chapter 1

Define Success, Clarify Expectations

Battle or Journey?

If you are like most of my clients, you are in a delicate state right now. The word "cancer" may have brought up other past experiences, fears or lingering pains. I am acutely aware of this, and have a huge amount of compassion for the battle that is likely going on inside of you right now. In order to help you begin this journey, it is important to honestly frame the situation we are starting with. I'm going to use a word that might feel a little difficult here. Not because that will be the outcome of your pet's cancer journey. It very well may not be. But because I know the word "cancer" leads most people to think about death. When you receive the diagnosis, you are met with conversations about prognosis and life expectancy. I know thinking about death is painful. I know you don't want to. But I also know, at least some level, you already are thinking about it. The word "cancer" puts your mind there.

So with both care and honesty, I want to bring some gentleness to this topic.

Western medicine has conditioned us to approach medical care as a battle of sorts. We fight death at all costs. Death is considered a failure, but it is not. Death is a part of life. It is the other end of our journey. No doubt losing someone we love is painful. But it isn't helpful to add feelings of having "failed" to the experience.

Everything in our life changes. Everything.

Life is a series of cycles. Every year has spring, summer, fall and winter. Every day has a morning, day, evening and night. Birth, living and death are all phases in the cycle of existence here on this planet. Just as the darkness of night gives way to the light of morning and a new day, every death is also the herald of a new beginning. If you believe that we are more than just a physical body, death is a new beginning for the being who transitions. Even if you don't believe that now, you might later. Or you may not.

In any case, your pet's death, whenever that eventually comes – hopefully a long time down the road – will be a new beginning for *you*. It will be the beginning of a new stage of your life: life after your pet. So the question is, what will you do with your one precious life? How will you make the most of the opportunities in front of you?

Mindset is a huge key in allowing you to engage with life's challenges in a way that can create beauty where at first there seems only pain. "The War Against Cancer" is one of the most destructive mindsets promoted in our journey of caring for the cancer patient. If you do have this mindset, I encourage you to let go of it. It focuses on the disease, not the living being. And, most unfortunately, it creates a belief, whether acknowledged or not, that if we don't cure the cancer we have lost the battle; that we have failed.

How, then, can we define success? I see it like this: We have problems. We identify solutions. We implement those solutions. We do our best with the resources we have available to us. We honor our individual goals for life. And we focus on healing. If we want to do the absolute best we can do, we focus on whole-being healing. We focus on *living*. We focus on Life. That process includes you, the pet parent, because you are your pet's whole world. You are the Sun in your pet's universe.

Expectations

So how do you engage with a healthy plan of action in the midst of the emotions you are undoubtedly experiencing now?

What you want may not be what happens. There are a lot of reasons for that. And there are many reasons that statement brings up resistance, anger, denial, hopelessness, despair or any number of difficult emotions. Having expectations sets you up for disappointment. But you also need aspirations, and hope, in order to have the motivation to take action.

Hope is essential for you to move forward. There is a delicate balance between action and surrender. We must take empowered and intelligent action. And we must then let go enough to allow life to unfold, and be able to entertain the possibility that there may be more to the picture than we can see now.

That is one of the trickiest parts of our human life, so much so that it has been addressed in every authentic spiritual tradition since the beginning of time.

I will get back to this later in the book. For now, I just want to plant the seed of awareness that there may be more for you in this experience than you can imagine, or are willing to believe from your current vantage point. There can be peace in that knowing, especially when you balance it with intentional action and loving compassion, both for yourself and the precious being in your care.

Rather than being focused on whether the cancer is cured or not, I invite you to focus instead on the experience of the *journey* you are creating for you and your pet.

First, take the steps along the path that you decide serves your primary goals best. Then, shift your focus to appreciating every moment, and learning as much as you can along the journey. This creates an opportunity for you to take positive action, growing through this process and making the most of the time you have together.

So, how do we define success?

What if instead of defining "success" as whether the cancer is cured, redefine "success" as whether you did the best you could to live well, and to help your pet to live well.

- "Did I do my best with the information and resources I had at the time?"
- "Did I honor my life and the life in my care to the best of my ability?"
- "Did I allow myself to find peace and my own healing through this journey?"
- "Did I learn something about myself?"

These all come down to one question: "Was I able to turn this challenge into an opportunity for growth?" If the answer to this is yes, then you will be at peace. What if you could accept that as "success"? Would it help you?

Success

I invite you to embrace this new measure of success as you create a path forward for you and your pet: Living well and transforming this challenge into an opportunity for growth. In this book, I offer you a way to walk that path of peace with your pet after their cancer diagnosis, should you so choose: Body, Soul and Spirit.

I have helped others walk this path; it is the most rewarding thing I do. I have many patients who are so much more than pets. I often think those furry beings are like little angels who have come into their person's life to help them in certain ways. If you are reading this book, it is likely that you have that relationship with your pet too. They are part of your family. There is a depth and potential to that relationship. Even though you feel it deeply, you may not yet fully understand the gifts they are bringing you.

I have had many clients come to me and say that they feel their pet brought them to me. The journey with their pet started a process for them to make important positive changes in their own life. This is really why the work I do in my integrative veterinary oncology practice can be so rewarding. As a result of the journey, many people are brought to greater levels of awareness about what they can do for their own healing – all through seeking healing for their pet.

One such client, Rachel, came to me when her dog Buddy was diagnosed with splenic hemangiosarcoma, an aggressive type of cancer. I knew when I met them that their bond was more than "ordinary." Rachel often says she knows Buddy brought her to me. Here is her story of healing and growth in her own words.

Rachel's Story

Cancer. A diagnosis that nobody wants and a journey that nobody would willingly choose. I remember feeling as though I was drowning in heavy grief, great overwhelm, and the unshakable fear of the unknown as I anxiously absorbed all of the information about our aggressive, terminal diagnosis.

I was confident in my ability to follow the robust and thoughtfully curated cancer treatment protocol, but I had one big question that I never had the courage to ask. My burning question was, "How do you do cancer? How do I do this?"

I won't pretend to be an expert in navigating such a delicate and difficult experience. But, I knew that whatever was to come for us,

I wanted what was best for Buddy – for his body and for his spirit. His wellness would be at the forefront of every decision I made until the moment he took his last breath. I wanted to carry the weight of the diagnosis so that he did not. The only thing I knew how to do was to love him – and I committed to loving him through it.

While I knew we would receive expert oncology care, I was not aware of how much more Dr. Bannink had to offer. In the trenches of a cancer diagnosis, at a time when I had completely lost my way and could have been swept away by despair, she offered a glimmer of hope with an Ensofic Reiki healing session. It was my greatest desire that the little time I knew we had left be filled with comfort, love and joy, despite the undeniable challenges we faced, and there was nothing I was not willing to try.

My skepticism diminished as I experienced firsthand the wave of calm and deep relaxation from the healing sessions – relaxation that we both had been so desperately craving but hadn't been able to access. On some of our hardest days, the Ensofic Reiki offered deep calmness and grounding for us both. I was grateful for the support to find my way back when I was lost in the chaos, and I remain grateful that Dr. Bannink was able to provide this for us.

I did not anticipate just how impactful this would be. It served as a reset for me, allowing me to navigate the rest of our journey from a more grounded and centered space. While I couldn't change our circumstances, I was able to change how we walked through them together. I was able to carry the heavy weight of the prognosis and make difficult decisions rooted in deep love instead of desperation and anxiety. This is my greatest hope for all pets and their parents, and why I share my story. I know how difficult this season is, and I know what an honor it is to love them all the way through it.

My only regret is that I did not embrace the other offerings sooner. Caught up in the overwhelm of a terminal diagnosis and navigating all that comes along with that – the stress and worry, the symptom scanning, creating joy in each day, managing herbs/supplements/ other treatments, anticipatory grief to name a few – while focused solely on my most precious friend, I didn't think I had the space to do one more thing, and I really didn't know how much it would actually help – so I waited.

While there is nothing easy about the journey through cancer as a pet parent, I realize now that the practical and tangible takeaways from the classes and other healings I pursued later would have immediately helped us to navigate it with more ease – which ultimately would have helped Buddy, something the clouds of grief hadn't initially allowed me to see.

I continue to lean on the community and tools I have gained from these offerings as I navigate the polarities of hope and grief. I am profoundly grateful to have had these resources to find grace on the hardest days of our cancer journey and to find my way back in life after loss – something I wasn't sure was possible.

It is a blessing that Buddy didn't know the weight of what we were facing and that I could hold that for him. It was my mission and my honor to carry that weight and love him all the way through. How grateful I am that this is how we "did cancer."

It's difficult to articulate just how much my life has changed as a result of these classes and healings with Dr. Bannink. Healing that

I sought for Buddy but didn't know I needed for myself. I am a completely different person now and I barely recognize the version of me that existed before my life activation – another healing that my mind didn't understand but my heart felt was important. My life is better – even after great loss. And if that is possible for me, it certainly is for you too.

I have walked through open doors into opportunities that welcomed me with grace when I was previously met with great inner resistance. I found the courage to let go of things and people that were no longer good for me. I have been able to quiet my mind and connect in more meaningful ways, living life from my heart instead of my head. Most profoundly, though, I was met with love and hope when I truly wasn't sure if that existed anymore.

So, while I sought out Dr. Bannink for her expert care of my precious friend on his hardest journey, I firmly believe that Buddy actually chose her for **me** *– his final gift divinely orchestrated to ensure that I would be OK long after we said goodbye. I continue to carry that love and watch it ripple out into all that I do.*

I hope Rachel's story will inspire you to entertain and embrace the bigger picture as you embark on your own journey through cancer with your pet and kindle an understanding that you and your healing are important as well. It can be helpful to know that sometimes the ultimate healing manifests in ways we don't expect or even know to hope for when we are starting on the journey.

CHAPTER 1 CHECK-IN

Let us take a pause here to check in. After reading Chapter 1, how would you define success on this journey, at this point? (Knowing that this might change as you read more and as you continue down the journey with your pet.) Pause and sit with this. Some questions you might consider:

1. How can I make the *journey* the best one possible?
2. What would that mean to me? What would that look like?
3. Other than "curing cancer," what other measures of success can I connect with right now?

Here are some examples to get you started on your own list

a. Focus on improving quality of life for you BOTH.
b. Laugh: Bring games, fun and playfulness into the treatment protocol.
c. Relax daily and enjoy each other without distractions.
d. Prioritize family connection time with your pet, like walks and playing games.
e. Focus on empowering actions you can take.
f. Learn to be more in the present moment.
g. Learn more about the power of diet in health and healing.
h. Appreciate life in a new way.
i. Have gratitude for the things you do have.
j. Take steps to improve your own health and well-being.
k. Learn more about yourself, your potential and your power.
l. Learn to love yourself the way your pet loves you.

Chapter 2

Identify Your Treatment Goals

Before we dive in, we must start at the beginning. Any plan requires a firm foundation on which to build a clear path forward and guide future decisions. The first step is to clarify your goals. The ultimate goal is to do what is best for your pet, given the diagnosis and within the abilities and resources available to you. What that looks like is different for every situation, which leads to other goals.

Everyone has different goals and, therefore, a different idea of what "success" looks like. Having clearly defined goals will help you make decisions when your emotions and stressors feel intense or overwhelming. As you move forward, you can come back to your goals to help you remember what is most important to you. Staying true to these goals will also help you feel more at peace about your decisions in the future.

- What is your primary goal? In other words, what is MOST important to you?

- What are your secondary goals? In other words, what is important to you but not as important as your primary goal? There may be many things here. Make a list and prioritize them 1–10.
- What are you willing to sacrifice to achieve those goals?
- What are you not willing to sacrifice?

Before you read further, I invite you to make a list of the above points. This list will change over time; it might change soon as you read further in this book. Don't overthink things right now. Just write what first comes to you. It is good to take stock of where you are now. There are no right or wrong answers – and we will revisit these later.

Examples of Treatment Goals

Now, let's take a look at some examples of common treatment goals. Cure and palliative care, or "comfort care," are two ends of the spectrum. In between these two are middle-of-the-road goals, aimed at slowing the cancer growth in order to extend good quality life. Integrative care is another more common goal that is gaining attention. This involves combining conventional "standard of care" treatments with other treatment modalities usually termed "alternative medicine," or nonconventional medicine. Let's explore each of these.

1. Cure

Maybe your primary goal is "cure." Many clients come to me with this goal. The important question to engage with at this point is whether – within the context of the realities of your pet's current situation, stage of disease, type of cancer, other confounding factors, and the resources available – this is likely. Consider the following questions:

- Has a cure been identified?
- How likely is a cure?
- What is the course of action recommended to achieve that?
- Do you want to do that?
- Are you able to do that?

This is where working with a board-certified veterinary oncologist can be very helpful as you explore all your options. They will be able to give you the most comprehensive and accurate picture of what conventional medicine has to offer. A board-certified veterinary oncologist is a veterinarian who has undergone rigorous specialized advanced training in cancer treatment. They can advise you on surgical, chemotherapy, pharmaceutical and radiation treatment options. They will also be able to share with you what kind of responses are typically seen, potential side effects, the cost of those treatments, and typical survival times with these types of medical interventions.

For them to give you the most accurate information, additional testing is needed to determine how advanced the cancer is in the body and what areas of the body are affected. These are called "staging tests" and may include biopsy, bloodwork, thoracic radiographs, abdominal ultrasound, CT or MRI, or other specialty testing. This is very valuable information to help you with initial treatment decisions and to decide how aggressive you would like to be. It will also help you objectively decide, based on accurate information, whether you are interested in pursuing conventional medicine treatments for your pet.

While a few board-certified veterinary oncologists such as myself have pursued extensive post-graduate training in Chinese herbal medicine, as of the time of this writing there are very few actively incorporating this in clinical practice. If you are lucky enough to be able to work with an integrative veterinary oncologist, this can open doors to other modalities that can be used alongside conventional treatments. If not, please respect that medical oncology training does not provide any actual training on herbal medicine use, and very few supplements are promoted in the conventional medicine treatment paradigm.

You would not go to your podiatrist and ask them how to treat your kidney problem, because that is outside the scope of their training, expertise and skill set. Similarly, to receive educated advice in herbal medicine options, it is necessary to consult a veterinarian who has both training and experience in the use of herbal medicine for cancer patient care.

I have seen cancer remission using herbal therapies, but this is very patient and cancer-type dependent. An honest and ethical practitioner will never promise you a cure. If you are interested in this approach, in order to receive the best guidance based on science, tradition and clinical experience, my advice is to work with a licensed veterinarian who:

1. Has a direct relationship with your pet. This means they have seen them and know all the details of their diagnosis and current health condition, as well as other medications and supplements they are receiving, and why. This is called having an established client-patient-veterinarian relationship.
2. Has advanced herbal therapy training and experience with herbal therapy prescribing for cancer patient care, or whatever modality you are interested in exploring for your pet.
3. Is willing to work cooperatively and collaboratively with the care team you want to build. This also holds true for your veterinary oncologist.

2. Integrative Oncology Care

The National Cancer Institute has defined integrative oncology as "a patient-centered, evidence-informed field of cancer care that utilizes mind and body practices, natural products and/or lifestyle modifications from different traditions alongside conventional cancer treatments. Integrative oncology aims to optimize health, quality of life and clinical outcomes across the cancer care continuum and to empower people to prevent cancer and become active participants before, during and beyond cancer treatment."[2]

Many cancers we see in veterinary medicine are not considered curable with conventional treatments. We can often achieve remission, meaning the cancer is no longer detectable with the tests we have available to us. But it is not cured because, over time, the cancer eventually returns.

In my clinical experience, in these situations it is often possible to achieve longer remission durations and survival times with an integrative oncology care approach. In my practice, alongside conventional cancer treatments, I utilize a combination of dietary interventions, Chinese herbal therapies, select nutraceutical supplements, acupuncture, energy medicine, lifestyle changes and mind/body/spirit approaches to support the family unit in navigating the cancer journey. This approach can not only increase survival time, but also optimize quality of life by improving energy level, normalizing appetite and minimizing other age-related quality-of-life issues like arthritis pain.

Principles of Combination Cancer Therapy

The principles of combination therapy in cancer treatment are to combine anti-cancer treatments that do not have overlapping toxicities in order to effect greater tumor control.

Iggy's Story

While all of the stories I am sharing in this book are examples of integrative care, Iggy is a great example of what a treatment approach relying most heavily on nonconventional treatments can sometimes achieve.

Iggy came to me at 6 years of age after surgery to remove his spleen due to a bleeding tumor. He was diagnosed with an aggressive cancer called hemangiosarcoma. His parents did not want to pursue chemotherapy for him, given the prognosis of about 6 months, and instead opted for a natural medicine approach after his surgery. They lovingly cooked him a balanced, fresh-cooked diet and elected a Chinese herbal therapy protocol. Iggy's hemangiosarcoma never returned, although he eventually developed oral melanoma many years later. While we were able to manage that successfully for a time, he eventually succumbed to the melanoma at almost 12 years of age, while the hemangiosarcoma was still in remission.

While Iggy is an outstanding example of survival and not all patients do this well, the average survival time I see with this natural medicine approach after surgical removal of the spleen is over one year, offering hope for this common and aggressive disease as oncologists and researchers continue our work to find better and better solutions.

3. Slowing Disease Progression

In cases where a cure is not expected or not realistically possible, or the path to "cure" is not chosen, I often recommend shifting treatment goals toward turning your pet's cancer into a chronic disease. This simply means focusing on halting the progression of the cancer so that it does not reach the point of affecting their quality of life. If your pet is not yet feeling sick from the cancer, this can be a good option. Sometimes it is possible to slow or halt the growth of the cancer so that they can live a comfortable life even with the cancer still present, or not "in remission."

This is also the option we move into in certain situations where pets turn out to be unusually sensitive to the conventional treatments being administered, and do not have the desired quality of life while receiving them. Fortunately, this last scenario is rare. But I have counseled clients to move into this treatment focus in some cases, because I believe strongly in prioritizing quality of life.

With this goal, combining multiple treatment approaches in an integrative oncology care plan can often help us reach this goal more effectively than with conventional cancer treatments alone.

Ancient medicine systems, which I will refer to as "traditional medicine," include systems such as classical Chinese medicine, in which I am trained. Traditional medicine systems have always understood healing as the restoration of *balance* in the body. With this approach, we are looking at the body as a whole, not just at the cancer itself. In other words, traditional medicine systems historically looked at the being affected by any illness from the perspective of the ecosystem in which that illness developed. In the case of cancer, this would mean not only considering the cancer itself, but the environment that allowed the tumor to grow in the first place.

Using the analogy of a garden, after killing the weed (with surgery, radiation or chemotherapy), you would then tend to the soil, making it a less hospitable environment in which any seeds still present could sprout and grow. Traditional medicines like herbal therapies have their strength in addressing the ecosystem, or the soil, while conventional medicines excel in extracting the weed.

In cases where the weed cannot be extracted, or when surgery, radiation and chemotherapy are not elected, we can turn our attention to the soil. This can make it harder for the cancer to thrive in the body, and in some cases halt its growth.

Modern Western medicine is beginning to move into this mindset more with the study of something called "epigenetics." Very simply, epigenetics explains how factors like behavior, environment, toxins, diet and stress can alter which genes in the DNA are switched "on" or "off." This can affect health and certain diseases like cancer development and progression. Cancer development and progression can be influenced by supporting changes in the ecosystem of the body to be less friendly to cancer growth and altering the signals that trigger gene expression.

Epigenetics is a huge topic outside the scope of this book. Just know that there are herbal, dietary and pharmaceutical ways to accomplish this, to name a few – and these each work in slightly different ways. This is the main way we can intervene to make it harder for the cancer to grow and survive in the body, allowing us to slow cancer growth, or even halt it. In a sense, you can think of it like making the cancer go dormant. It is still there, but it isn't growing.

Remi's Story

Remi is a great example of what can happen when we are able to make the cancer go dormant and stop its growth.

Remi was referred to me at 10 years of age for end-of-life comfort care. He had been diagnosed with anal gland adenocarcinoma that had spread to the lymph nodes, for which his family did not want to pursue aggressive treatment. The lymph nodes and the anal gland tumor were very large, so surgical removal was not an option. While his family initially expected only to discuss options to alleviate pain and discomfort, we discussed treatments that I had seen successfully halt the progression of anal gland carcinoma for meaningful periods of time. We were able to resolve his main quality-of-life issue of elevated calcium and stop the growth of his cancer for three years with Chinese herbs and zoledronate infusions.

4. Palliative Care or "Comfort Care"

Palliative care means care that focuses on alleviating pain and supporting comfort without the goal of directly treating the cancer. There are many reasons you might elect palliative care for your pet:

- When the cancer is so advanced that there is very little we can do to remove it or halt it.
- If your pet is very old, and aggressive treatment is deemed not to be compassionate or in their best interest.

- If your pet has other medical issues that prevent us from being able to treat the cancer aggressively and still maintain quality of life.
- If it is very difficult for you to administer medications to your pet at home.
- If your pet experiences such extreme anxiety when being handled or traveling to the veterinary clinic that treatment is not possible or not kind.
- If you or your family are dealing with severe mental/emotional challenges, your own health concerns or caregiving for someone else, and are therefore limited in what is realistically possible to healthfully handle or pursue.
- If treatment, even though desired, is financially out of reach.

Technically, palliative care means we only focus on managing pain and discomfort, not slowing cancer. However, I often combine these, as many herbal therapies and acupuncture treatments can accomplish both. In certain situations conventional treatments like "palliative radiation" may be an option to alleviate cancer-related pain without the goal of cure.

Some people feel very peaceful and certain about this goal from the start. Some people feel guilty about choosing this course of care. There is no such thing as right or wrong. Sometimes being aggressive with treatment is a less loving decision than shifting focus to supporting your beloved companion through the stage of end of life, and providing a healing, loving environment for you both as you walk the sacred path of life transition.

Barny's Unexpected Comeback

Barny's story shows how palliative care improves comfort and quality of life.

Barny was diagnosed with high-grade T cell lymphoma of the spleen and intestines and he was very sick from the cancer by the time I first saw him. His parents were extremely dedicated and decided to pursue an integrative chemotherapy protocol.

Despite our best efforts, his quality of life never improved and his cancer failed to respond to treatment, showing early signs of drug resistance. Because the cancer was progressing and his quality of life was poor, ten weeks after diagnosis we elected to stop chemotherapy as a compassionate measure. We shifted our focus instead to doing our best to support quality of life, and elected an aggressive herbal therapy protocol along with a balanced home-cooked diet and acupuncture treatments. To our surprise, he slowly improved. While his cancer never went into remission, the clinical signs he was experiencing from the cancer resolved, and he lived another nine months with a good quality of life, until the very end when the cancer progressed again.

What treatment approach is best?

Only you and your veterinarian can decide that. I will go into more details on treatment options in Chapters 5 and 6 to help you navigate these waters. In the end, the best decision is the one that will allow your pet the best life possible within your treatment goals, and the one that will allow you to have the most peace possible when you eventually say goodbye. Remembering we are all here for a short time, we can focus on the quality of life lived and the moments we are able to enjoy together on this journey of life. Your pet gives you so much and they may be one of your greatest teachers: on love, on acceptance, on living in the moment, and on making the most of every day. The best treatment approach is the one that honors that bond, their best interest and your love for them.

CHAPTER 2 CHECK-IN

Make a list of your treatment goals.

1. What feels most important to you right now?
2. What is your primary treatment goal? (Pursue a cure? Comfort care? Something in between?)
3. What are your secondary goals? In other words, what is important to you but not as important as your primary goal? There may be many things here. Make a list and prioritize them 1–10.
4. What are you willing to sacrifice to achieve those goals?
5. What are you not willing to sacrifice?

Examples of Treatment Goals

1. **Cure:** Attempting to completely eliminate all cancer.
2. **Integrative Oncology Care:** Combining conventional treatments with nonconventional treatments such as mind/body practices (for you), natural therapies, acupuncture, diet and lifestyle modifications in order to optimize health, quality of life and clinical outcome.
3. **Slowing Disease Progression:** Focusing on halting progression so your pet can live comfortably, while the cancer still present, for as long as possible.
4. **Palliative Care:** Focusing on alleviating pain and discomfort, without the goal of slowing tumor growth or decreasing tumor burden.

Chapter 3

Create a Stable Foundation

The better able you are to cope with the cancer diagnosis, and the more peace of mind you have, the better quality of care you will provide to your pet. The single most important factor for you in both coping and caring will be your trust in the doctor(s) you are working with.

There are many correlations between veterinary oncology and pediatric oncology. Cancer affects the well-being of the entire family unit. From studies evaluating peace of mind in parents after a cancer diagnosis in their child, we know that over 75% of parents experience low peace of mind and that low peace of mind, anxiety and depression can persist for many years, regardless of treatment outcome. Additionally, stress contributes to impaired problem-solving and coping mechanisms. This distress relates to difficulties in parents' ability to adapt to the oncological situation, and being overwhelmed in the management of daily life. Their ability to cope with the cancer diagnosis is correlated with the quality of care they are able to provide.[3, 4]

Those studies show most parents are changed by the cancer experience, even when cure is achieved and the future is bright. When looking at long-term peace of mind, complete trust in their oncologist at the start of treatment was significantly associated with higher peace of mind five years after diagnosis.[5]

Trust in the doctor you work with is therefore paramount to your being able to navigate this journey with more peace and less suffering. Trust is a necessary component of every relationship. Being able to trust the oncologist or veterinarian you work with through this journey is important to your well-being, and to your veterinarian's ability to help your pet to the highest of their capacity with all the resources and skill sets at their disposal.

If you don't trust your veterinarian or veterinary oncologist, that must be addressed in order for you to optimize your own well-being and allow you to provide the level of care I know you want for your pet.

Trust can be a tricky thing for many people. "Betrayal wounds" from past experiences, or social conditioning encouraging distrust, make it a substantial challenge. This is a subconscious influence in many cases. You may not even be aware of how it is affecting your thoughts, emotions and behaviors.

Below are some common reasons I have seen people struggle with trust in the cancer setting over the last two decades. Do you see any of these tendencies in yourself? How can you address these in a healthy way, so they are not acting as obstacles to creating the best experience for you and your pet?

Three Common Reasons for Distrust

Difference in treatment philosophy

If you only believe in natural medicine and do not feel comfortable using pharmaceutical drugs, for example, it doesn't make sense to work with an oncologist or primary care veterinarian who has no training in those treatments. Without training, they cannot provide an educated assessment based on understanding that treatment modality. They can only offer their opinion.

A conventionally trained veterinarian will not have answers to your questions about Chinese herbs, for example. Seek out someone who has expertise in the treatment approach you are interested in pursuing, so you are able to receive an educated assessment of whether those treatments are likely to be beneficial, and to what degree. You may need to build a care team with people who are comfortable working collaboratively to provide a treatment plan, building the experience to support you and your pet in the way you wish to be supported.

A word of caution: There is such a thing as "too many cooks in the kitchen." I do see clients who seek out the opinions of every possible person they can. They then have so many conflicting recommendations – and so many treatments and supplements – that they become confused and overwhelmed, which becomes detrimental to their pet's care. My best advice is to work with as few people as possible. Choose ONE doctor for conventional care and ONE doctor for alternative care.

Too many treatment philosophies muddy the waters and overwhelm your pet's system. More is not better.

Ideally, if you can find one doctor who has training in all the modalities you are interested in, stick with ONE. As of the writing of this book, there are very few integrative board-certified veterinary oncologists, but we do exist. Interest is growing. And I do have clients who have traveled across the country to work with me.

Not wanting to believe what you are being told

This is a difficult and very real phenomenon. Doctors never enjoy delivering bad news. But part of our job is to present you with an honest assessment of the situation. Doctors can certainly be wrong, and their perspective may be colored, like every human, by their training, personal experiences and beliefs. But for most cancers in veterinary medicine, we have decades of clinical experience – and, in many cases, clinical data providing very helpful statistics to guide treatment decisions. This data is a valuable resource for us to help you rise above the emotionality of the situation, and make informed decisions about how you would like to move forward.

I tell my clients, "We use statistics to make treatment decisions, then we forget those and we do our best every day. **Your pet is not a statistic,** and even if there is a 5% chance a treatment may work, if it works for your pet, that is all that will matter for you. However, it is important to understand the choices you are making."

A veterinary oncologist will be the best person to advise you on conventional cancer treatments, the potential side effects, the outcomes, and associated average survival times. They will most likely not have any educated information about alternative medicine treatments. They may offer their opinion, and it may be a very emphatic one. But opinion is not the same as educated experience.

There is a period of time in which the shock of the diagnosis, emotional overwhelm and anticipatory grief will make it difficult for you to think clearly. That is a normal result of stress. You will also be going through the stages of grief. You will experience anticipatory grief. That is all normal. You may find yourself getting stuck in one of the stages of grief, such as denial, anger or bargaining. That is also common, but it isn't helpful to your ability to move through this journey in the best way. This is also important to be aware of and understand, because it impacts how you are able to receive and process information from your veterinary care team. I will circle back to this in a moment.

Believing the cure for cancer is being intentionally withheld

This has become a more and more prevalent obstacle to trust in the medical profession over the past decade, and has become a much more common phenomenon lately. As of the time of this writing, this is an unfortunately common social dynamic that fosters suspicion and breaks down the client-patient-veterinarian relationship. This is especially true with the advent of "Dr. Google" and the extensive amount of differing opinions, perspectives, motivations and propaganda in the media at large and, specifically, in many social media groups. Emotional manipulation is the main method used to direct your attention and capture your beliefs.

In this day and age, it is common for people to feel inundated with misinformation, fostering suspicion and breaking down all sorts of relationships. This ultimately breaks down society, which requires healthy relationships to thrive. I am not here to tell you what to believe, and it is not the focus of this book to explore this in more depth. I bring this up because it is important for your well-being to understand what dynamics are influencing your mental and emotional state, and your ability to connect with a medical professional who can help you navigate this journey.

I can't tell you how many clients I have that experience unnecessary fear, anxiety, guilt, doubt, anger or shame because of comments and "advice" from individuals on social media platforms. While these groups may have started with good intentions, it is not unusual to find they devolve into unhelpful drama factories, either intentionally or unintentionally promoting distrust in the veterinary care team. I have also even seen comments disregarding the medical advice being recommended by the patient's veterinarian. This is not only potentially harmful to your pet, it is not supportive of your mental and emotional state. If you find yourself relying on these groups for support, understand that not all patients are equal, and not all cancers are the same. What works or doesn't work for someone else's pet may not apply to your pet's situation or circumstances. Additionally, if you are being criticized or shamed for decisions you are making with your veterinary care team, you are not being supported – you are being bullied. You should seek sources of information that are balanced, properly moderated, supportive and compassionate.

I encourage you instead to educate yourself without divisiveness. It is important that you feel able to explore options that are important to you. Just know that your veterinarian is not in it to withhold an effective treatment from your pet. If you do feel that way, look for someone else you can trust, and work with or address this within yourself. See if you can find a healthy balance of empowered and healthy skepticism while respecting the experience of the veterinarian you choose.

Creating a stable foundation for this journey is an essential step that will bring greater peace of mind and support both you and your pet as you move forward. A veterinary care team you trust, and a treatment plan that you feel is aligned with your goals, will be a centering place you can return to as the journey unfolds.

CHAPTER 3 CHECK-IN

Have you positioned yourself well to be in a good place to support your pet through this journey? Once you have identified your treatment goals, find a care team you trust and who understands those goals.

Here is a quick checklist to help you identify places you can adjust to create a more stable foundation for the journey ahead.

Have you put together a small but mighty veterinary care team?

If you have more than one veterinarian, the others on your team should complement each other's skill sets and be comfortable working together. At most, you might have:

- your primary care veterinarian
- your veterinary medical oncologist
- your veterinary surgeon
- your veterinary radiation oncologist
- your alternative medicine veterinarian

There may be exceptions to this, depending on your pet's needs.

Do you trust and respect all the veterinarians with whom you have chosen to work?

If you answer no, I recommend taking positive steps toward effectively addressing this for yourself. Remember, this is not about trying to change other people. This is about identifying what you need to do to help you move toward your treatment goals.

Chapter 4

Assess Your Resources

The next step is to honestly take stock of your current resources and future potential resources. While this can be difficult to consider, it is vital to create a plan that allows you to maintain a safe and healthy environment for both yourself and your pet.

What are your resources? Resources include: money, time, emotional bandwidth, energy, physical ability, and professional and social support.

- What is your **financial** budget for pet care and treatment?
- How are you doing emotionally and mentally? Are you able to access resources to support you **mentally and emotionally** if you need that?
- What kind of **time** do you have?
- Do you have **physical** limitations that may influence the type or intensity of care you are able to provide? And if so, do you have people to help you?
- Do you have **people** to support you?
- Do you have a **veterinarian** you feel you can trust?

Planning Financial Resources

Can you afford the treatments required for your stated goal? It is important to consider what you need in order to be able to meet at least your basic financial needs to afford housing, transportation, food and health care for yourself and your human family. While pets are important, they are not more important than the people in your life. And they are not more important than you. This is a more common struggle than you might think.

Do you *want* to afford the treatments? Some people have the financial resources but have other commitments that are of higher priority. This is both a "reality of life" and a personal choice and is ultimately your responsibility to determine. Your primary care veterinarian or veterinary oncologist can help you navigate the pros and cons, but this is something that ultimately comes down to you and your priorities.

There are many emotions that often come up around financial decisions.

Mental/Emotional Support

Finances are a huge source of stress for many people. I want to share some common struggles that arise around the issue of money because, in my experience, these are a huge source of mental and emotional stress for many people. They can erode your ability to enjoy the precious time you have with your pet, and the beautiful echoes of their life after they are departed.

If you are feeling any of these, you are not alone. Sometimes just bringing awareness to your reactions, and understanding that these are common, can help loosen their hold and power over you. This will give you space to process these emotions in a healthier way, either on your own or with a licensed mental health professional. You can let them move through you so that you can arrive at a reasonable decision for yourself, your pet and your family.

Anger

This often manifests with thoughts like "Treatments are so expensive. It isn't fair." Or "Treatments should be given for free." This anger is often directed at another person such as the veterinarian you are working with, a family member, a group like the medical profession in general, or even God.

Anger is sharp. And it eats you up from the inside, making a challenging situation more painful and amplifying your suffering. This is sometimes difficult to combat or remedy without a lot of personal awareness or someone to help you look at things differently.

Guilt

Guilt can arise either from not being able to afford a treatment or deciding to do a treatment you have mixed feelings about. This is so common that I spend a lot of time helping people navigate this. It is, quite honestly, one of the main reasons I am writing this book. Guilt destroys your ability to enjoy life, and it is often difficult to resolve after the fact. It keeps you from having peace about your decisions. And it keeps you stuck in past decisions that cannot be altered.

Having clarity about what is most important allows you to focus on what you CAN do. This empowers you to make the most of life and every day, while also acknowledging that we all sometimes make mistakes. Those mistakes are also learning opportunities. Having a care team you trust goes a long way in supporting you in making the best decisions for you and your pet – and having peace around those decisions.

Establishing a clear path forward that empowers you to take the right positive action to create healing opportunities for both yourself and your pet is the best way I have found to make life fulfilling, and to connect you with hope and self-worth.

Shame

Shame often accompanies lack of financial resources and, sometimes, the worry that your lack of ability to afford a treatment will cause others to think you don't care for your pet. This is extremely common, and often results in reluctance to be honest with your veterinarian about the realities of your financial resources. If they don't know, they cannot help you explore options that are financially within reach. And they cannot guide you in navigating how to move forward with your pet's care within the realities you are facing.

If any of these feelings are overwhelming or adversely affecting your quality of life on a regular basis, working with a licensed clinical therapist or counselor can be a huge support for you and your loved ones – particularly if you work with someone who understands the impact of the human-animal bond.

They can help you process these emotions in a healthy way, and learn techniques to redirect and calm your thoughts and emotions.

There are also other things that can complement appropriate psychological intervention, which we will get to later in the book. Now here is an exercise to help you with this process.

EXERCISE: Imagining to Find Clarity and Peace

In my experience, guilt is often the most problematic lingering emotion when what we want and what has happened do not align. Knowing you did the best you could for your pet within the context of your resources, and what you desire for their life, can be a soothing balm as you navigate the waters of grief. This is true both for the grief that naturally arises after their cancer diagnosis (anticipatory grief) as well as the grief after their eventual passing, whether from cancer or another cause.

For clients struggling with a decision, I often recommend the below exercise and ask them to notice how they feel in each scenario. This is a way to explore which course of action provides the most peace, and the least guilt. You can think of this as an exercise in imagination: "What if."

If you are emotionally able to engage with this exercise without becoming overly distraught, it can provide some perspective, and help you arrive at a treatment decision that brings you a measure of peace, regardless of the ultimate outcome of the journey. As with everything in this book, be gentle with yourself. If this feels like too much, don't do it.

1. Make a list of the treatment options you are considering.
2. Put yourself, just for a moment, at the end of your pet's life.
3. Now, working with the first item on your list, imagine you pursued that course of treatment and are now saying your final goodbye. It will always feel sad and difficult. But do you feel any regrets about doing or not doing something? Can you feel at peace within your goodbye knowing that you did what you felt was best for them and for you both?
4. Repeat this for each item on your list.
5. Which option allows you to feel the most at peace about the choice you made?

I find that, for many people, this exercise can be very helpful in negotiating difficult decisions where the outcome is uncertain. For example, some people will tell me they need to feel like they have tried everything possible within reason, and then they will know they did everything they could. That would bring them peace. If they don't, they will feel guilty for not trying it, and will always wonder if the outcome would have been different had they done something else.

Some people will tell me they don't want to try everything, because what is most important is that their pet has the least amount of intervention possible and is comfortable. They would feel extremely guilty if there were any side effects from the treatment and would feel more at peace having focused solely on comfort.

Working with a veterinary care team you trust is very important here. They will be a good, objective advocate for your beloved pet as you are in deep emotional waters. They will help you know when your pet is suffering, and when they are not. For most of my clients, this is always their primary concern.

Emotional attachment can be very hard to release, and there are situations in which people are unwilling to say goodbye, even when their pet is experiencing extreme pain and suffering. It is in these situations that trust in your veterinarian is particularly essential. It will allow you to be able to accept information that is hard to hear so that they can help you stay true to your primary and secondary treatment goals. This is the main key in decreasing the likelihood of guilt after your pet's passing, rather than feeling "I waited too long" or "I didn't do enough."

Other Resource Considerations

Time

Time is an important consideration as you plan your treatment approach. For example, are you going to be able to take time off work to attend appointments? Can you create time windows for your pet's care that still allow you to honor your other commitments? The time commitment will be very individual, based on your pet's needs and the kind of cancer they have. Your veterinarian will be able to help you understand the time commitment.

Physical Limitations

This is not an overly common problem. However, it bears mentioning. For example, if you have a large dog that requires major surgery, such as limb amputation, you may need to consider post-surgery care. Are you able to physically assist them in standing as they learn to re-adjust how they walk? Can you help them in and out of the house to go to the bathroom? Do you have stairs they will need to navigate? Maybe you need to get a ramp to help them get in and out of the car.

People to Help You

Do you have friends or family who can help you with appointments or other resource needs? Emotional support? Assistance administering medications? Preparing food? If you are planning to travel, do you have options for pet care with people who are willing to administer the medications your pet might need?

A Veterinarian You Trust

I addressed this important issue at the start of the chapter. Every veterinarian commonly faces these issues with clients, and we can help you navigate decisions that help you find a balanced path forward, within your means. We do care. We can share our perspective, but we cannot make the decision for you.

CHAPTER 4 CHECK-IN

Checking in with your goals: Have they changed?

Here is a good place to revisit your goals from the previous chapters.

- What is your primary goal? In other words, what is MOST important to you?
- What are your secondary goals? In other words, what is important to you but not as important as your primary goal? There may be many things here. Make a list and prioritize them 1–10.
- What are you willing to sacrifice to achieve those goals?
- What are you not willing to sacrifice?

Part I Takeaway

Preparing for the Journey

Acronym for your foundation: T.E.A.M.

TREATMENT GOALS: hope
EMOTIONS: acceptance
ASSESS RESOURCES: strategic action and allocation
MENTAL POSTURE: trust

Treatment Goals

- Focus on hope.
- Get clear about your treatment goals.
  - Cure
  - Slowing disease progression without intent to cure
  - Palliative (comfort care)
  - Integrative Care

Emotions

- Be aware of how your emotions may affect your ability to make decisions.
- Be aware of how the information you consume influences your emotions.
- Pursue responsible and effective support if you need help managing your emotions to help you have the best experience.

- Balance intentional empowered action with acceptance. Having a plan you feel good about will help with this.

Assess Resources

- Allocate resources strategically, based on your treatment goals.
- Plan ahead to help you prepare.
  - Finances
  - Time
  - Mental/emotional capacity
  - Physical demands

Mental Posture

- Trust allows you to have peace through the journey.
- Your ability to trust the advice you receive from your care team is important.

PART 2

THE PHYSICAL BODY

An Empowering Approach to Healing

As we develop a broader view of health and healing, we are empowered to take an active role in treatment, recovery and thriving. Treatment then becomes not a "battle against cancer," but about how to optimize life.

This focus is emotionally healthier for both veterinarians and pet parents. Ultimately, it is a more effective approach to healing and support of the human-animal bond. It allows us to focus on wellness, rather than focusing on disease. And, in the end, the quality of the life that is lived during the journey of cancer treatment is almost always improved.

More Than Medicine

There are a great many things we can do to care for our physical body. "Prevention is the best medicine" could not be more true, especially when it comes to cancer. Once the body becomes out of balance and develops illness or disease, many factors contribute to a successful and complete recovery to a healthy balance state. Medications are definitely one method we have to correct imbalance. That is what our Western medical system is primarily designed to provide.

That isn't the whole picture, though. Beyond tumor-directed treatments, steps can be taken to support the body's natural defenses against cancer and tools are available to make the body a less cancer-friendly environment. Going a step further, it is also important to consider how to improve the quality of life lived after a diagnosis of cancer. This is one of the benefits of integrative medicine. Combining the strengths of the Western biomedicine paradigm with traditional medicine paradigms, which have a long history of supportive lifestyle and natural medicine therapies, we open the door to improving outcomes for our cancer patients.

Research is growing on how diet, vitamin levels, exercise, lifestyle, stress, herbal medicines and acupuncture impact the development of and recovery from cancer in humans. We now also know that the health of the gut microbiome, which is strongly affected by diet, may impact individual responses to conventional cancer therapies like chemotherapy and immunotherapy. This research on lifestyle and botanical medicine from the human literature informs new science-based perspectives in integrative veterinary care, and inspires veterinary research into these aspects of health and healing.

I will be the first to admit that my medical training promoted a bias for me personally. Although I was open-minded, and while I definitely believed it could help cancer patients feel better, I did not believe acupuncture or Chinese herbal medicine could treat cancer. In my residency days, I had a strong bias against accepting that acupuncture and herbal therapies could slow tumor growth or shrink tumors.

To be fair to my training, this belief was heavily influenced not only by what I was told in veterinary school and my medical oncology training, but also by the overwhelming number of clients giving herbs to cancer patients I was treating based on internet searches and information. Not one of them was getting better. In most cases, these were single herbs or simple herb combinations, touted as "detoxifying" agents – and general claims that the supplement could "cure cancer."

In my case, rather than telling all the clients who came to me for guidance that "herbs don't work," I realized I had no actual basis of education for that statement. I had not researched herbs to any degree, and had pursued absolutely no training to support my understanding of the limitations or applications of herbal traditions. While I had no solid information on which I could recommend herbal therapies for cancer treatment, I also did not believe that the ancient herbal medicine traditions that have existed for thousands of years could continue to persist and be in use if they were not helping people.

I decided to get training and discern for myself. My initial rationalization was that I could, at the very least, help alleviate some of the suffering my aged patients were experiencing as a result of being old and having cancer, such as low energy and arthritis. I pursued acupuncture certification, and for my acupuncture internship hours I studied with Dr. Steve Marsden, who is not only a veterinarian but also a naturopath with a Master of Science in Oriental Medicine.

He encouraged me, despite my skepticism, to try a few specific Chinese herbal formulas and see what my experience was. As I applied my Chinese medicine training to prescribe the formulas properly to the appropriate cases, I began to see results that surprised me. When I had my first cancer patient who experienced tumor regression with herbal therapies alone, where conventional treatments had failed, my beliefs began to shift. My direct experience no longer supported the belief that "herbs can't shrink tumors."

I also saw cases in which the herbs did not work. So, equally, I did not hold the naive view that "herbs cured all cancers." Nor did I believe that just because one patient experienced results, the same treatment would work for all patients. Cancer patient care is a nuanced art. Now, with decades of clinical experience behind me, I have thousands of patients who have taught me that every patient is different and requires a patient-specific approach.

During my residency, when I first embarked upon my acupuncture training and began exploring herbs for my clients seeking guidance on alternative therapies, I scoured PubMed and the university library. Back then, there were far fewer research articles than exist now. But they did exist, even then. That time in my life marked a shift into the realm of integrative cancer patient care.

It also taught me valuable life lessons:

- I don't, actually, know everything. That's ego talking.
- There is always more to learn.
- Other people's opinions are not a sound basis upon which to base my beliefs.
- Opinion and personal biases are not strengths; they limit us.
- There are very intelligent people doing important things not accepted by mainstream society, or even our modern medicine paradigm. That doesn't necessarily mean they are ineffective.
- A healthy dose of skepticism paired with humility, the openness to learn, and the willingness to be wrong is a powerful combination that opens new doors and moves us forward.

Most importantly, I lived the experience of the statement you will hear me make over and over: Information doesn't change beliefs; experience does.

Every breakthrough began with someone asking, "What if we could do better?" Progress depends on those with the courage to question, to explore, and to imagine possibilities others have yet to see.

Chapter 5

Conventional Western Biomedicine Therapies

The focus of this book is to assist you in navigating the cancer journey with more ease and to empower you. The arena of conventional cancer therapies is evolving quickly, and new advancements in research change the face of cancer therapy yearly. My best advice for you to receive up-to-date information on the current Western medicine options is to schedule a consultation with a board-certified veterinary oncologist. They will be able to best advise you on the treatment options for your pet.

Here, I aim to give you a very brief overview of the basics of conventional anti-cancer therapies, so that you have some idea of the types of treatments available and what to generally expect from them. This is important because many clients come to me with misconceptions about what cancer therapy involves and what it means for quality of life. There are even still some primary care veterinarians who will advise clients against seeking out conventional oncology treatments, based on outdated information.

Below are some of the more commonly used conventional medicine cancer therapies explained very simply. Your oncologist can provide a more detailed explanation, with specific considerations pertaining to your pet's unique situation. This is just meant to give you an idea of the kind of treatments available. It is not intended as an exhaustive list, as treatments are constantly evolving.

Maximum Tolerated Dose Chemotherapy

With this type of therapy, high doses of chemotherapy drugs are used with the aim of damaging the cancer cells directly so that they undergo something called *apoptosis* – programmed cell death or "cell suicide." This type of therapy works best for rapidly growing tumors.

These drugs are injections or oral chemotherapy agents given in intervals, usually weekly to monthly. Side effects vary based on the drug being used. The most common side effects are low white blood cell count, nausea or diarrhea. The severity of these in most pets is nowhere near what humans often experience. It is common for people to have a lot of fear around giving chemotherapy to their pets, due to experiences they have had with their human family members, loved ones or themselves.

For most drugs, the drop in white blood cell count is most pronounced 7–10 days after treatment. With proper monitoring, these drops are rarely dangerous to your pet. If the white blood cell count falls below a certain level, your veterinarian may recommend antibiotics to prevent infection while their counts recover, typically for only about one week. Platelet count can also decrease with some drugs. This also rarely causes bleeding problems, but it is important to monitor as the future doses of chemotherapy agents may need to be altered. Your veterinary oncologist will monitor these numbers closely in order to make appropriate adjustments to your pet's medical care. If your pet is experiencing treatment delays due to these issues and you are working with a veterinarian trained in Chinese herbal therapies, there are herbal formulas I have found very effective at supporting blood counts to minimize the impact of these side effects.

Nausea and diarrhea, if seen at all, usually occur 2–5 days after treatment and resolve with a bland diet and medications at home within 2–3 days. Poor appetite is more common than vomiting. Your veterinary oncologist will discuss with you the specific risks associated with the chemotherapy agents being recommended for your pet and provide medications to treat these side effects if they occur. Acupuncture and herbal therapies (see later section) can also be very helpful in preventing and treating these side effects.

Metronomic Chemotherapy

Metronomic chemotherapy is a strategy of chemotherapy administration that uses low doses of oral chemotherapy agents at regular intervals, often daily. This type of treatment aims to inhibit the process of new blood vessel formation, or angiogenesis, that tumors need in order to supply nutrients needed to grow. This treatment can also make it harder for the tumor to hide from the immune system by changing certain immune responses involved in protecting tumor cells from immune system attack.

Angiogenesis, the process of new blood vessel formation, is important in both the growth of the main tumor and the ability for cancer cells to spread and develop into tumors at distant sites, a process called "metastasis." It is a popular topic in the forefront of current cancer therapy, and much research is being done on targeted therapies designed to inhibit the ability of tumors to form their own blood supply.

Targeted Cancer Therapies

These are aimed at blocking or inhibiting specific signaling molecules or pathways that are involved in the growth of specific types of cancer. Tyrosine kinase inhibitors, like Toceranib, are one example of this type of treatment. There are many of these types of drugs currently in use and under development in human cancer treatment. Many of those same drugs are being used in our veterinary patients now as well. Side effects are typically mild and vary depending on the drug. These are sometimes combined with high-dose chemotherapy protocols.

Immunotherapy

This type of treatment administers cancer "vaccines," for example, which are designed to help the immune system recognize cancer cells and clear them from the body. Many cancer vaccines have been developed, but at the time of this writing, very few have proven benefit in veterinary medicine. Other types of immunotherapy generally increase immune surveillance and boost anti-cancer immune responses. There are some herbal therapies and supplements that can also improve anti-cancer immune responses to augment conventional therapies.

Repurposed Drugs

This refers to the use of drugs that were originally developed to treat non-cancerous conditions. A simple example of this would be non-steroidal anti-inflammatory drugs like carprofen and piroxicam. These drugs block COX-2. Overexpression of COX-2 has been demonstrated in a variety of veterinary tumors: transitional cell carcinoma, osteosarcoma, melanoma, prostate adenocarcinoma, canine oral squamous cell carcinoma, canine renal carcinoma, canine nasal carcinoma, canine mammary carcinoma, and feline mammary carcinoma. Other examples of repurposed drugs evaluated for cancer in pets are Auranofin and Naltrexone. Auranofin, a gold nano-particle originally used to treat rheumatoid arthritis, has some research in veterinary medicine for treatment of osteosarcoma in dogs after amputation and chemotherapy.[6] Naltrexone, a drug originally used to treat opioid addiction, administered in low doses has been evaluated in the management of mammary carcinoma in dogs.[7]

Surgery

Physically removing the tumor from the body is the best way for most tumors to be treated. Some can be cured this way. Others are not cured, but removal decreases the number of cancer cells remaining in the body in order to make it more likely that follow-up treatments will be effective or helpful. For most surgeries, recovery time is 10–14 days. Even with large surgeries, like those requiring removal of an organ from the belly, dogs and cats bounce back quickly. While it is hard for many people to think about, amputation is also surprisingly well tolerated in most dogs and cats who are otherwise healthy and who are not severely overweight. Those with severe arthritis or other mobility issues are not good candidates for amputation.

Radiation

Radiation is a treatment where high-energy beams are aimed at a tumor in order to damage the cancer cells so that they die. There are a few different types of radiation therapy in use in veterinary medicine. This is most commonly used to kill remaining cancer cells when surgery was unable to remove all the cancer from an area. It is also used for decreasing tumor size in tumors that cannot be surgically removed, or to treat pain associated with bone tumors. Radiation does cause side effects to the normal tissue surrounding the tumor. Stereotactic radiation therapy is a type of radiation therapy now available in veterinary medicine that allows higher doses to be delivered to the tumor with less normal tissue side effects. Radiation requires general anesthesia to administer.

Electrochemotherapy

This is a treatment in which chemotherapy is injected along the surgical scar, followed by an electrical current to make the tumor cells more susceptible to the chemotherapy. This is a local treatment usually used after surgery to treat residual disease but can also be used as a primary treatment in certain situations. Side effects are usually limited to local tissue reactions from tumor die-off or mild local inflammation. This requires general anesthesia to administer.

Conventional medicine provides many good options for dealing with aggressive cancer and is considered the standard of care in the United States and many other countries. It is important to understand and consider these options when exploring a comprehensive care protocol for your pet, as there are many types of cancer in which these will significantly improve survival time or the ability to control disease for longer. It is also important to understand the true risks of these therapies, as many people have preconceived ideas about the severity of side effects, which may not be accurate and could result in overlooking an option that may actually help your pet experience less pain and live longer. Many of these treatments can be incorporated into an integrative treatment plan with the interventions discussed later in this book.

CHAPTER 5 CHECK-IN

Western Medicine

- Strong in addressing acute, catastrophic physical illness.
- Many lives have been saved with advances in physical medicine, surgery and biomedicine.
- Cancer is often viewed as an invader, taking over host resources.
- Treatments like chemotherapy and radiation are aimed at eliminating this invading presence. These treatments can be particularly useful in rapidly progressing tumors, as they kill rapidly dividing cells. However, they also affect normal tissues such as bone marrow and the cells lining the gastrointestinal tract. While these treatments have their place in cancer treatment, they are not always a guarantee of cure.
- Drug resistance is a common threat to the effectiveness of these therapies, which is why research looks for ways to overcome or prevent drug resistance.
- Scientists are looking to herbal compounds for their potential to prevent multiple drug resistance and are making promising discoveries.

Beyond Surgery, Chemotherapy and Radiation

- **Metronomic chemotherapy:** This type of treatment aims to inhibit the process of new blood vessel formation, called angiogenesis, that tumors need in order to supply nutrients needed to grow. This treatment can also make it harder for the tumor to hide from the immune system by changing certain immune responses involved in protecting tumor cells from immune system attack.
- **Immunotherapy:** This type of treatment administers cancer "vaccines," for example, which are designed to help the immune system recognize cancer cells and clear them from the body.
- **Targeted therapies:** This type of treatment is aimed at blocking or inhibiting specific signaling molecules or pathways involved in the growth of specific types of cancer.

These treatments are becoming more widespread in human oncology, and we do have options available for veterinary patients. Many, however, can be limited by high cost, are not widely available, are still in the clinical trial phase, or may not be effective in dogs and cats due to differences in their bodies or tumor types.

Healing is not the application of a remedy;
it is the restoration of balance.

Chapter 6

Alternative Medicine

Everything that does not fall under the umbrella of conventional medicine is relegated to the "alternative medicine" category. This includes a very wide array of interventions that is beyond the scope of this book. My alternative medicine expertise and clinical experience is in Chinese herbal medicine, acupuncture and metaphysical healing, so these are the modalities to which I am qualified to speak and provide information about.

I have been a veterinary acupuncturist for almost 20 years, as of the time of this writing, and have a Graduate Diploma in Veterinary Chinese Herbal Medicine through the College of Integrative Veterinary Therapies (CIVT). I have completed a number of advanced Chinese herbal training courses with Dr. Steve Marsden, one of the leading experts in veterinary Chinese medicine. I have also pursued advanced training in metaphysical and energy healing techniques in the Mystery School lineage of King Salomon through the Modern Mystery School, which works tirelessly to ensure these ancient teachings maintain their purity as they are disseminated to the public.

I actively maintain my certification and pursue regular continued education to ensure I stay in integrity with the teachings.

In my clinical experience, these treatments can each provide meaningful contributions to a whole-being care protocol, either as adjuncts to conventional treatments or as primary interventions when conventional treatments are not elected.

The Vision of a Unified System of Healing

One important aspect to consider as we begin our exploration into the subtler realms of healing is that conventional Western medicine cancer treatments, at this time, focus primarily on physicality. That is our training and the primary arena of Western medicine. This approach is a relatively recent phenomenon and is not the case in many well-established, ancient and, what I am calling here, "traditional" medicine paradigms, where there is a more open acknowledgment of the various dimensions of our whole-being. These include not only mental and emotional aspects, but also energy, Spirit, Divine energies and our connection with the world around us.

Before I open this line of thinking as we get into the main focus of this book, I want to be very clear that I do not intend to imply that modern medicine is "bad" and traditional medicines are "good" – simply that they are different. There is a place for both if we consider the strengths of each. I, after all, incorporate both into my patient care and would not do so if there were not benefits to each. For example, while there is all manner of controversy over the ills of modern medicine in some circles, it is true that due to the discoveries and advances in modern medicine, humans no longer die of certain things that were once common causes of death.

Yes, we are now dealing with different challenges and side effects of pharmaceuticals, which have caused real quality of life problems for real people and pets. That does not discount that an honest look into the state of medicine now shows we are much better equipped to deal with severe, sudden-onset, life-threatening emergencies than we were 100 years ago. Modern medicine, however, is poorly equipped to address chronic diseases. That fact is more and more apparent as we see the growing emergence of degenerative conditions.

Some might say that is because we are living longer, which is true. That, however, glosses over the fact that many young people are experiencing chronic diseases at a rate never seen before. Traditional medicines have a paradigm that lends itself more strongly to addressing and correcting chronic diseases, and the true traditional medicine systems have always acknowledged that there is a nonphysical aspect to our health and healing. Some called that energy. Some called it Spirit. But this was the realm of the true Shamans and metaphysical healers, who worked with Divine universal energies. And they did affect healing.

It was really during the 19th century movement separating science from spirituality that the spiritual realm got relegated to a completely different place, categorized by the "scientists" as myth, folklore and fantasy at best, and ignorance at worst.

"Pseudoscience" is now a word that people who seek to discredit those who work in these other realms often use as a weapon to defame and discredit other approaches.

But I wonder, if we could unify our understanding of health and healing once again, leveraging the strength of our scientific advancements with traditional wisdom that is still aligned to the correct energies, what results might we achieve in greater well-being, with each taking its proper place in our health and healing and being appropriately recognized for what it can and cannot achieve? I think this would only strengthen our outcomes in cancer patient care – and my clinical experience supports this.

I look at cancer, fundamentally, as a chronic disease, which can have acute manifestations. In other words, it can seem to "come on suddenly." In the acute setting, Western medicine shines. But we need better answers for re-establishing an environment in the body that is in balance to better address long-term outcomes and quality of life.

Acupuncture

There is still, apparently, a pervasive myth circulating in the veterinary community that cancer patients should not receive acupuncture because it will make the cancer grow. This is categorically untrue. I am not sure where this idea came from, other than the fact that cancer often worsens, unrelated to the intervention. So perhaps fear, rather than fact, was the originator of this story. There are now numerous clinical studies demonstrating the benefit of acupuncture in supporting cancer patients, and it is commonly incorporated into integrative cancer care programs throughout the world.

The rationale I have often heard used to back up this belief is that acupuncture increases blood flow, which feeds the tumor. However, if one understood the traditional system of medicine and how acupuncture is prescribed and delivered as a whole-body treatment, it would, firstly, not be necessary to put a needle directly into a tumor. Secondly, for decades most of the research in acupuncture (and Chinese herbal medicine, for that matter) was not translated into English. This resulted in statements from Western doctors and veterinarians such as "no research exists," which is often not true. It may be true to say "I don't know of any research," or " the quality of the studies does not withstand rigorous scrutiny." But that is not the same as "there is no research" or "acupuncture makes cancer grow."

Robust research did not exist in English until relatively recently, but acupuncture has been in use in the East for over 3,000 years. Chinese medicine practitioners in the Eastern world have centuries of experience using acupuncture in animals, not to mention humans. It is an arrogance of attitude that would presume that only Western science has merit or that because the Western medical community has not embraced a particular therapy, or deemed it worthy of clinical investigation, that it does not have the potential for benefit in cancer patient care.

Some ways acupuncture may support cancer patients:

- Improve appetite
- Decrease nausea and vomiting
- Resolve diarrhea
- Increase energy levels
- Decrease pain
- Restore the proper movement of the stomach and intestines
- Improve blood counts
- Support kidney and liver health
- Minimize anxiety or anxious behavior

Herbs

As acupuncture was my gateway to experiencing the power and potential of properly prescribed Chinese herbal formulas in managing cancer patients, I am including these modalities here in the Physical Body Health section. These modalities can be explained from both a physical science biomedicine viewpoint and from the perspective of Energy, if one approaches them in the way they were traditionally developed and conceptualized.

When we are working with whole herbs especially, there is a certain vitality that is brought to the healing that comes from the living organism from which the medicine was constructed. We can feel this vitality when we eat food fresh from the garden, and for that reason, in veterinary medicine we are often encouraged to put the category of herbal medicine into the specialty of nutrition.

The problem with that is herbal therapies are actually prescribed based on the patient, and we have not generally approached nutrition in that way, other than specific nutritional recommendations for extreme imbalances that include organ function failure, like kidney failure and liver disease. Lumping the complex system of traditional herbal medicine into the category of nutrition does not do justice to the nuanced prescribing systems, or the fact that these treatments can restore health and are not, beyond general wellness supplements, appropriate for every animal. Nor is every herbal cancer formula appropriate for every pet with cancer.

For many skeptics, herbal medicine and even acupuncture are still today often lumped into the realm of "woo-woo" medicine. This is a bit surprising if one remembers that many of our chemotherapy and pharmaceutical drugs had their origins in plants. There is also now a plethora of research on herbal compounds that are being mined for their potential development as anti-cancer drugs and as sources for compounds to prevent the development of chemotherapy resistance.

Companies would not invest in this kind of research if there was not sufficient evidence that these traditional herbal therapies, from which the researchers are pulling subjects of study, did not show promise of effectiveness from a biomedical standpoint. Fortunately, as we begin to wake up, challenge our cultural and medical biases, question beliefs, and become a more global society, this negative bias is shifting.

Since my early herbal medicine and acupuncture days of 2005, and especially since 2017, the number of research studies evaluating Chinese herbal therapies and acupuncture has skyrocketed. Now, there are thousands of research articles on herbal medicine and cancer patient care published in the English language. In brief, these studies show that acupuncture can alleviate pain and fatigue, reduce chemotherapy side effects, minimize bone marrow suppression from chemotherapy treatments, improve sleep, and assist in brain function, all while also being associated with low risk of adverse effects. As research continues, the number of gold-standard, large-scale, randomized, placebo-controlled clinical trials will continue to inform the best use of acupuncture for cancer patient care.[8, 9, 10, 11, 12]

Jason's Story – From Hopeless to Helped

Jason is one of those patients who will stick with me forever. Not because he lived "forever," but because he was tangible evidence that the integrative treatments I was offering made a difference in the lives of both pets and people.

Jason had been diagnosed with osteosarcoma, the most common type of bone cancer in dogs. It is an aggressive type of cancer with a survival time of one year with the "standard of care" conventional treatment: amputation and chemotherapy. After amputation he had been undergoing Carboplatin chemotherapy treatments at a different specialty cancer center. Although Carboplatin is usually well tolerated, he was one of the few patients who really had a lot of significant side effects. His appetite and energy level were so poor after the first few treatments that his family was struggling with a euthanasia decision due to a lack of options to relieve his suffering and restore good, quality life. After discussing this with their primary care veterinarian (who knew I was trained in Chinese medicine), she suggested they make a consultation with me to see if I could help him prior to making an end-of-life decision.

When I saw Jason, he was barely eating and his energy level was so low that he wasn't doing any of the things he used to enjoy. This had been going on for a few months.

I treated him with acupuncture and an herbal formula called Liu Jun Zi Tang. Over the next few days his appetite markedly improved and his energy level dramatically increased. We were able to bring his quality of life back to normal, which provided both him and his family additional precious time that they did not think they would have. And, importantly, that time was excellent quality time.

Over the course of my career I have seen many patients in "hopeless" situations like this, who have been told there is nothing more that can be done. I often used to wonder what I could do for these patients if they had been sent to me at the beginning of their treatment, rather than after failing every conventional medicine intervention. This is commonplace for alternative medicine practitioners.

Now, after over 20 years in specialty practice, I am in a position where clients seek out appointments with me at the start of the cancer journey. Because of this, I have countless stories of patients who have far exceeded their life expectancy, and years of clinical data in real patients to back this up.

What I often wonder is, given the power of the human-animal bond, what could we achieve if the humans who are sharing this journey with their pet actively and eagerly pursued their own healing, and were open to prioritizing the well-being of the whole family unit? Still today, the number of clients who are willing to put energy into their own well-being is far lower than I would like to see. Although they are often willing to do "anything" for their pet, I often wonder why it is so hard for us humans to prioritize our own healing.

I have personally witnessed acupuncture, herbal medicine and energy healing infuse vitality into patients' failing bodies. The same is true for people. While I am not licensed to treat humans in this way, there are many who are. I encourage my clients to also prioritize their own health and healing by working with qualified professionals. What I *am* trained to do is help humans access greater levels of spiritual health. That is an arena I am passionate about. I have seen firsthand how it can create positive ripple effects that support improved physical, mental and emotional wellness. This is the topic we will dive into later in this book.

The traditional systems of medicine always defined health as "balance," not as lack of disease. We would be well served to explore this idea in the modern setting and, taking it further, to ask better questions. Such as: What are the true components of whole-being balance? If we take our lead from the ancients and the wisdom keepers, physical, mental, emotional and spiritual are all intertwined. Neither is independent of the other. Each contributes to our state of balance. And if one is neglected, the others eventually suffer.

When you are exhausted, anxious or feeling a lack of peace and purpose, your pet will pick up on this and may even mirror you. When you are tending to all these aspects of your wellness, your pet will benefit as well. When you have more energy, they will enjoy your elevated mood and increased capacity to play, exercise and enjoy life with them. When you are feeling more mentally and emotionally at peace, have more physical vitality, and are more connected to the spiritual aspects of life that support you in feeling a greater sense of meaning and purpose, your pet will be the happy beneficiary of your improved state of balance.

CHAPTER 6 CHECK-IN

Chinese Herbal Medicine: Many herbs are adaptogens, immune modulators and anti-inflammatory agents. There is much research emerging on the anti-cancer effects of herbal compounds and some Chinese herbal formulas. Many herbs, for example, have shown the ability to block tumor progression pathways and angiogenesis (the process of new blood vessel formation).

It is important to work with a veterinarian trained in these modalities who can help you make sure you are avoiding adverse drug-herb interactions. Not all interactions are bad. There are some herb-drug interactions that may be beneficial, improving the action of either treatment alone.

Acupuncture: This is an important option in palliative care, supporting appetite and energy and minimizing side effects from conventional treatments or the cancer itself. There are many veterinarians trained in acupuncture.

Things You Can Do

Acupressure:

- Massage the muscles along the spine. The area right in front of and behind the last ribs is especially helpful for appetite and digestion.
- Massage the forehead, between the eyes, to calm your pet.

Chapter 7

Food as Medicine

This book is all about empowering you to make the best decisions for you and your pet. This means focusing on what you can control, and a key area of this is the food you feed your pet. Let us look at the research, the options and my recommendations based on more than 20 years of clinical experience working with pets.

A clean, balanced, healthy diet is the cornerstone of health. The food we consume provides the building blocks of our body and provides resources that are used to heal and maintain a balanced body ecosystem. This is well-recognized in human medicine.

Though there are many differing opinions on what type of diet might be best for the cancer patient, the common thread weaving through all opinions in the human medicine circles is that fresh, clean food is ideal, and processed food promotes cancer development. This has been published in many epidemiological studies over the past few decades.

- The typical Western diet, which includes a relatively higher amount of ultra-processed foods, has been consistently identified as increasing cancer risk and higher risk of death from other non-cancerous causes.[13, 14, 15, 16, 17, 18]
- Ultra-processed food consumption of a mere 10% increase in dietary intake has been associated with increased cancer risk in humans.[19, 20, 21, 22, 23, 24]

There is no logical or rational reason to assume animals are less susceptible to the adverse effects of processed food. While diet change may not be within reach for everyone, it is one of the important factors we have a measure of control over in our journey to improving well-being for both ourselves and our pets.

It has been well-recognized by science that diet affects cancer risk, and it is estimated that at least one-third of the most common human cancers can be prevented by a healthy diet.[25, 26, 27]

There is also evidence that dietary interventions are one powerful way we can intentionally impact tumor progression in animals.

- Research in animal models has shown that cancer development, growth and response to therapy are impacted by diet timing, caloric content and macronutrient composition.[28, 29, 30, 31]
- When done without causing malnutrition, calorie restriction by 15–30% reduces tumor development and slows tumor growth.[32, 33, 34]

- Numerous studies in animal models have also shown that cycles of fasting may make tumor cells more susceptible to cancer therapies.[35, 36, 37]
- New research also suggests that dietary factors may influence response to cancer immunotherapy (cancer vaccines).[38]

In clinical veterinary practice, strategic feeding can be a challenge because of the human component. People project their emotions and their relationship with food onto their pet, and are often resistant to limiting treats or controlling calorie intake. Common reasons for this resistance are the belief that their pets will not be happy without their special treats, or that restricting their food intake will cause suffering in some way. Other clients are open to this type of intervention. Additionally, the media is inundated with widely varying opinions on the best diet for pets with cancer.

In my experience, this has made the diet topic highly emotionally charged and traumatic for many clients, initiating feelings ranging from confusion and overwhelm to guilt and blame. It can, on the other hand, be an empowering place to intervene if we focus on where we DO have control and keep our eye on the big picture.

Rather than getting tied into the latest feeding trend and engaging in divisive arguments about whether there is published research to support a benefit in feeding fresh, clean foods to veterinary cancer patients, I recognize that common sense should not be disregarded merely because there is not a randomized, double-blinded, placebo-controlled clinical trial proving that what is generally considered a healthy diet is, in fact, healthy. Humans and animals have been eating for millennia without this scientific validation. It is only recently that industrialization has presented new factors such as extruding and heavy herbicide application to crops, a change that has seen a parallel increase in cancer rate in both pets and people.

Having said all of this, below is the way that I, at the time of this writing, approach the diet conversation with my clients and how I guide them in developing a feeding protocol that considers not only their pet's health, but the realities of their resources and their preferences.

A thorough presentation of the scientific literature on this topic is outside the scope of this book. Furthermore, new research is being conducted all the time, so that in just one year whatever nuances I may cite here may be refutable or refined with new research and an evolution of our understanding. It is up to you to stay abreast of the topics that interest you and make educated decisions about whether you believe my recommendations or wish to consider them. I will share here what over 20 years of clinical experience and personal relationships with clients who have been witness to the changes in their pet after diet change have demonstrated to me: Improved vitality, coat quality, and general quality of life, not to mention survival time, are results to pay attention to.

I recommend my clients focus on feeding a diet that has the least amount of carcinogens possible, and which is nutritionally balanced and optimized based on our current level of understanding, which is evolving all the time.

As of the time of this writing, there are chemicals in processed pet foods that are not healthy. The main ones are glyphosate, found in common weed killer, and AGEs (Advanced Glycation End products), which form when food is processed at high temperatures. A study out of Cornell University showed that dog and cat foods contained much higher levels of glyphosate than the FDA allows in human food products. Glyphosate level was shown to be associated with the plant component of the pet foods.[39] To avoid this chemical, you would need to feed a pet food that contains organic plant ingredients (hard to find) or is meat-based.

To minimize your pet's exposure to AGEs, you would need to eliminate foods that are processed with high heat, such as all regular hard kibbles. This type of processing is called "extruding." Additionally, if we are looking to feed the highest quality food possible, the starting ingredients should be at least food materials that are approved for human consumption.

I am very selective about the foods I recommend for my patients. What I look for is a well-balanced diet, minimally processed, that is fresh. In my clinical experience, I have not seen a huge difference between quality of life and vitality in pets fed a lightly cooked, clean, balanced fresh-food diet and those fed raw – although both can be done improperly, and not all pets do well with the same diets. I recommend working with a veterinarian who is educated on fresh, balanced diets if you are able to afford this way of feeding. Not everyone has the financial resources to do this. Fresh, clean food costs significantly more, just like the food you eat.

In my practice, the focus of our consultation is education so you understand the choices you are making and are able to make the best decisions within your means.

I have data from my clinical practice proving that, for some cancer types, fresh, clean, balanced diets, when used as part of the integrative protocol as I practice it (I can't speak to those results in others' hands), results in longer survival times compared to pets fed processed kibbles and canned foods. Data like this that shows correlation cannot tell us *why* that is the case. That requires further investigation. I am aware that making any kind of statement about diet invites heated debate these days. Nevertheless, this is what I see in real patients in real-life clinical practice, and it serves no one to deny that reality.

I have hope that as time goes by and we evolve our understanding of true healing, health and wellness that this will begin to become more widely understood by all facets of the veterinary community. Until then, as a pet parent, you must be aware that you may talk to 10 veterinarians and get 10 different opinions with associated justifications. I am not here to make other people wrong. We are all products of our training and conditioning and life experiences. You, reading this book, are no different. I am aiming here to share with you a plan for success that I have seen help thousands of pets now. An important ingredient in that recipe for well-being is good food.

Having said all this, it is of primary importance not to add feelings of guilt to an already difficult situation or exacerbate the stress you are experiencing. I have three strict rules that I offer to guide feeding decisions as we are formulating a feeding plan.

Three Rules for Feeding:

1. The food is nutritionally balanced to the best of our current level of understanding.
2. Your pet likes the food and eats it.
3. It does not stress you out. *Stress comes in many forms: time, money and relationships. If the food is adding to conflict and stress, it is not a good choice for our Whole-Being Wellness program.*

If any one of these guidelines is not able to be met, we must go back to the drawing board and adjust our feeding plan. Just like food you eat, fresh, real food diets are more expensive than highly processed food. Both a good-quality, commercially prepared, fresh food option or a properly prepared, balanced, home-cooked diet may be financially out of reach. Or you may need to sacrifice a nonessential expense to be able to afford this adjustment.

Commercial, processed, shelf-stable food is convenient, and fresh diets can be a time stress for many people. Home-cooking correctly, although often less expensive than purchasing a high-quality commercially prepared food, is more complicated than throwing some chicken, organic rice and carrots together. Home-preparing a properly balanced diet that will adequately support your pet can be overwhelming for a lot of people.

In these cases, the solution might be feeding half of the diet as fresh, clean food and the other half as high-quality processed food that is relatively lower in carcinogens. It might mean not changing the diet at all. Some of that depends on your pet's condition, and whether they have other concurrent health problems requiring special dietary restrictions. This is why it is important to work with a veterinarian who is both educated and sympathetic to what you are trying to achieve.

If you can meet the three rules, then you can optimize the power of food by feeding an ultra-clean, balanced diet free of carcinogens and chemicals, avoiding highly processed foods and treats, and even including some "superfoods."

- Organic foods are higher in micronutrients and macronutrients than conventionally grown foods, which will provide additional nutrition without added calories.[40, 41]
- Dogs fed a raw, meat-based diet were shown to have improved composite clinical health scores compared to those fed extruded kibble diets.[42] Fresh-cooked diets were not evaluated in this study.

Taking an Empowered Approach to Feeding

Conscious pet parents, like you, are expressing an increasing interest in feeding interventions for their pets after a diagnosis of cancer. This has resulted in a boom of information widely available on the internet from sources ranging from pet parents sharing their experiences to board-certified veterinary professionals, each vehemently defending their positions and opinions. There is no cohesive information and often it is cloaked in fear, blame and finger-pointing.

This all can lead to a situation in which anxiety, stress and financial distress can further decompensate an already fragile human emotional system that is trying to adjust to the recent diagnosis of cancer in a beloved pet, and the accompanying fear and worry. The number of pet parents coming in to see me who express significant fear and anxiety over the food they are feeding their pets has increased significantly over the years preceding the publication of this book. I can tell you, this is exceptionally heartbreaking.

For example, I had a concerned pet parent come in who was extremely distressed because she was afraid to feed kibble but couldn't afford to do a nutritionally balanced, fresh-food diet. Despite a lengthy conversation including diet options at her integrative oncology consultation the week prior, she had started feeding her dog a two-ingredient home-cooked meal, which was not remotely close to being nutritionally balanced, based on the recommendations of an online community.

When we discussed other options, she cried, sincerely concerned about putting her pet back on kibble, based on what she had been told by this "support group." Fortunately, because I checked in with her about her pet's diet at his visit, we were able to discuss other options that were financially feasible for her and better nutritionally for her pet, while not discounting her concerns.

Another scenario that I often see is that pets just won't eat what we would like them to eat. I had a kitty patient, for example, whose refusal to eat anything but a very limited array of processed foods was causing her "mom" significant anxiety. She really wanted to feed her a less-processed diet, but her kitty just would not accept the other balanced foods that were being offered. In these situations, a processed balanced food is comparably better than eating, for example, a diet comprised of 100% baby food. But finding a balance among the intense emotions arising from fear, including anxiety, guilt and blame, can be very challenging.

Overcoming Fear and Guilt

Many pet parents express that they feel that what they fed or didn't feed their pet caused cancer, or that by not changing the diet they are "killing" their pet. The first and most important thing to understand is that there is not one thing that causes cancer in every pet or person. And while it is intelligent to consider how we can use food as medicine, food is not by itself a singular cause of cancer, nor is it an independent cure.

It is true that chronic, low-dose exposure to carcinogens (many of which have been identified in processed foods, both human and pet) may be a contributing factor for cancer development. It is also true that certain nutritional deficiencies have been shown to contribute to cancer risk. It is, however, also true that many pets live a long life without developing cancer who have eaten a poor-quality kibble or diets of fresh foods that would be identified as nutritionally unbalanced, based on animal nutrition standards.

A balanced perspective is important when considering the best path forward.

Controlling What We Can Control

The environment we live in is much more toxic than it was years ago. This is likely one contributing factor to the rise in cancer we are seeing. Stressing over this is not helpful. But we can ask the question, "What do I have control over?"

Food is one of the things we can control. The relevant question in veterinary cancer patient care is ultimately not "Are chemicals scientifically proven to cause cancer in dogs and cats?" but rather "Is it medically harmful to limit exposure to known carcinogens when possible?"

The most basic way to shift into a place of empowerment is to change the question we are asking. Instead of "What should I NOT do?", a more effective approach would be to ask, "What CAN I do?" Within that question lies empowerment. And it helps us move away from making decisions based on fear and into an emotional atmosphere of making decisions based on positive action.

Hemi's Unexpected Cure

Sometimes we do absolutely everything we can and nothing touches the cancer. We don't get even a fraction of the outcome we wanted. Sometimes, in those situations, I can see something else is at play – a bigger picture for their person. The river of life sometimes takes us in unexpected directions. Our task, if we choose to accept it, is to learn to steer our ship, stay balanced and keep moving forward.

Other times, we see wonderful results! Every oncologist has their miracle stories. Hemi is one of mine. He is an example of the potential an integrative cancer treatment approach carries.

Hemi came to see me when he was just 3 years old. He was diagnosed with Diffuse Large B Cell Lymphoma, which has a median survival time of 11 months with standard of care chemotherapy (CHOP protocol), or 19 months with an integrative oncology approach in my hands. His calcium level was high, which is often associated with a less favorable prognosis.

Hemi's family understood the probabilities of his situation. They decided on a path forward and then focused on supporting him. They also had a strong network of support who helped them with his care and veterinary appointments. They had a team working together. Making his food; giving medications. Not everyone has that. They also had the financial resources to make that work.

His parents elected an integrative treatment protocol, adding a fresh, balanced, home-cooked diet, Chinese herbal therapies, acupuncture and supplements to his chemotherapy treatment regimen. With this type of treatment, once the chemotherapy protocol is finished, the herbal therapies and supplements are continued as a maintenance therapy.

Hemi finished his first round of chemotherapy and continued his herbal regimen and fresh, clean, balanced diet. He came in for regular lymph node checks to monitor his remission status. The average duration of first remission is about six months for most patients. Hemi stayed in remission for one year – the average survival time for this kind of lymphoma.

We restarted chemotherapy, but this time he had bladder complications from one of the chemotherapy drugs and we decided not to continue his chemotherapy treatments. The family's mom had just given birth to twins, and they chose to do what was necessary to realistically support the whole family. I can tell you it wasn't an easy decision for them to stop chemotherapy. Hemi was their first "son." When they decided to stop chemotherapy treatments, they accepted what that decision probably meant. And they stayed focused on loving him and supporting him with the anti-cancer lifestyle we had put together for him.

They continued his home-cooked diet, herbs and supplements for quite a while. Eventually, they stopped his herbs. Hemi stayed in remission from lymphoma for the rest of his life. He lived a love-filled life until he finally left the world at the age of 11 due to unrelated causes, almost eight years after his diagnosis of lymphoma.

Hemi is an uncommon example of a best-case scenario. Cure is not at all common for Diffuse Large B Cell Lymphoma, which is considered an incurable cancer – although I commonly see extended survivals in patients of mine that receive an integrative treatment approach. Hemi is a great example of the fact that probabilities are not always what happens. No one could have predicted he would enjoy the long and health-filled life he did. I certainly didn't know.

I always tell my clients, "I've been doing this long enough to know you never know. We just need to make the best decisions we can and then move forward doing what we are able to do."

10 Empowerment Strategies

1. Think Long-Term and Be Realistic

- Find a diet that you can realistically maintain long term.
- This includes understanding the realities of your finances, lifestyle, time constraints, other life stressors, and your pet's personality and willingness to eat certain diets.

2. Read and Understand Food Labels

- When seeking out commercially available diets, be sure to select those that are intended as a complete and balanced diet. Diets labeled for "intermittent feeding" do not meet AAFCO minimum requirements for a balanced diet. (AAFCO is an industry standard for minimum dietary requirements.)

- If you are interested in feeding a lower-carbohydrate food, you can calculate carbohydrate content based on the food label, because carbohydrate content itself is not required to be listed on the pet food bag. "Grain-free" foods are often still quite high in carbohydrates, especially kibble varieties.
- If you are interested in feeding a less-processed diet, look for one that indicates that low-heat processing methods were used. Cooked foods will be "slow-baked." Shelf-stable "raw" foods will be "air-dried," "freeze-dried" or "dehydrated."
- All foods, not just raw, should undergo processes and testing to address potential bacterial contamination. (Bacteria contamination food recalls have occurred with *both* fresh food and dry kibble foods, even when treated to prevent bacteria.)

3. Consider Supplemental Options

- There is a growing body of evidence in human medicine that supports the benefit of phytonutrient-rich foods in cancer chemoprevention and treatment, and the role of vegetable and fruit consumption in decreasing cancer risk.
- If you are unable to pursue a nutritional consultation to formulate a balanced, home-prepared, fresh-food diet, supplementing your pet's diet with a small amount of nutrient-dense foods (for example, broccoli sprouts, cruciferous vegetables or green leafy vegetables) or

administering carefully selected supplements may be a manageable way to provide phytonutrients that are not available in highly processed pet foods, and that have some evidence of potential benefit in cancer nutrition.

4. Educate Yourself

- Seek out accurate information and form your own points of priority in your pet's nutrition.
- Understand where the information is coming from and biases or agendas that may be influencing the information, so that you are able to make informed decisions based on the information you acquire.
- Bring your concerns about nutrition and your dietary goals to a veterinarian you trust to help you in the discernment process and assist you in making decisions about your feeding options within the context of your personal situation, and your pet's individual health priorities.

5. Focus on Well-Being

- Your pet's outward signs of well-being are a helpful measure to determine the impact of the nutrition they are receiving. Increased energy, good body condition, shiny hair coat and healthy skin are all good outwardly visible measures of overall wellness.

6. Clean Up Your Pet's Diet

- If you are concerned about ongoing carcinogen exposure and toxic stress, being mindful to limit chemicals, coloring and preservatives, as well as process contaminants (these are substances like acrylamide and heterocyclic amines, which are liberated during processing) can be helpful in minimizing the toxic load on your pet's system.

- Even if you are unable to feed all organic unprocessed foods, making more informed choices in pet treats and pet food options can improve the "cleanliness" of your pet's diet. While experts may still disagree about the role this plays in cancer prevention or treatment in dogs and cats, it is certainly not harmful.
- Be mindful that "clean," "natural" and "raw" are buzzwords for marketing strategies. These food label claims don't mean much in and of themselves. Do your research, consider the processing methods and ingredients used, and recruit your best common sense to help you determine if the food meets the "cleanliness" goals you have for your pet's diet.

7. Short-Term Perspective

- Understand that, short of severe nutritional inadequacies, most nutritional imbalances will not manifest in clinically significant ways until after many months of feeding an unbalanced diet. So if your pet requires or is only accepting certain foods that are not nutritionally balanced, don't panic. There is time to find a workable solution.

8. Engage with Healthy and Effective Support

- There are a plethora of resources and well-intentioned "support groups" for people caring for pets with cancer. The first thing to ask yourself is whether or not, in these support groups, you are actually feeling supported. If not, I suggest seeking out alternative resources that provide you with the emotional support that is helpful to you. Criticism, negativity and judgmental attitudes are toxic to your already stressed emotional system.
- Seek out kind people and information that focuses on empowering you, not scaring you.

9. Focus on Evidence That Is Not Emotionally Toxic

- Select information resources that focus on positive empowerment, compassion and understanding that is also grounded in evidence.
- Evidence may come from the veterinary literature or, because the veterinary nutrition and oncology professions in the United States have not recently placed priority on research and clinical trials to identify optimal nutrition for pets with cancer, information may, by necessity, be extrapolated from the human literature.

10. Make Your Well-Being a Priority

- Remember that the love and care you show your pet is the most important aspect to their well-being and enjoyment of life. They only know how they feel every day, and how they experience you. Finding a balanced approach to their care that allows you to feel good about what you are doing and minimizes avoidable stress is an important part of formulating an effective care strategy.

Your Well-Being

You are also an individual with your own medical history and health challenges. I am not a human nutritionist or functional medicine doctor, but it may interest you to connect with someone if you feel you need more assistance with this aspect of your own wellness program. Here I will offer some general considerations that apply specifically to supporting you as you walk this post-cancer-diagnosis journey with your pet. It is always recommended that you consult with a licensed nutritionist, functional medicine doctor or other trained professional to guide you in making specific medical decisions. You are always your best advocate. Educating yourself empowers you to also take control of your own health so that you can work collaboratively with your own health team.

Eat healthy yourself. This increases your energy and has been scientifically shown to decrease symptoms of depression and anxiety. When you feel better, you will be better positioned to navigate difficult decisions with less overwhelm, have greater vitality to enjoy the time you have with your pet, and will be better able to stay centered and balanced to be a stable caregiver during this time.

CHAPTER 7 CHECK-IN

Decide what you are able to do to make one shift toward a cleaner diet for you and your pet. You can both enjoy this adjustment and share the journey to supporting your bodies in this healthy way.

Starting Small

- Swap out one unhealthy snack or treat for one healthy one for each of you.
- For example, you might decide to replace your nightly potato chips with a green smoothie, and your pet's processed treats with cubed cooked chicken breast as treats instead.
- As you both partake of your new snacks, share a snuggle and some good pets as you have a chat about how these healthy foods are good for you and give your body the building blocks to become stronger.

All Out

- Maybe you are ready to make the diet switch altogether and really get clean with your eating and your pet's eating. Maybe you even start buying organic and healthier foods for your whole family.
- If you are ready for this level of commitment, transition gradually over 2–3 weeks to let everyone get used to the changes.
- Make sure you are feeding everyone a balanced diet.

- Remember that simply feeding your pet what you eat will not be adequate to provide for their nutritional needs, as they will require calcium and minerals as well as additional vitamins and possibly fiber to make sure they are getting what they need every day over time.
- As you are transitioning to this new clean eating routine, take joy in the preparation and plating of the food.
- Appreciate the hard work that went into providing it for you: the farmers who raised it, and the people who harvested and delivered it.
- Think about how this nourishing food will support your pet and your family to provide their bodies with the building blocks for healing and vitality.
- Maybe you even share meal times so you are all enjoying this food at the same time.
- And then go for a 20-minute walk with your dog afterward as you digest. Or snuggle with your kitty as you pet them and tell them three good things that happened for you that day.

Middle of the Road

- Choose somewhere in the middle. Maybe you aren't ready or able to go all out but you want to do more than a snack swap.
- You can consider feeding one meal a week as your "clean meal," or just swapping out 25–50% of your processed food consumption for cleaner options.

Esoterics

Esoteric means the hidden meaning underneath the surface. It is the deeper "why" underneath everyday knowledge and apparent reality. Esoteric wisdom is often called "hidden" wisdom. That isn't because it is secret or forbidden, only that it requires deeper contemplation and reflection because the meaning isn't obvious on the surface. It can, ultimately, only be experienced and felt. Esoterics can be thought of as the study and practice of accessing deeper spiritual knowledge that helps us understand who we really are, why we're here, and how to live in alignment with universal truths.

Chapter 8

Diving Deeper: You Are More Than Your Body

Taking care of the physical body is an essential Cornerstone to Whole-Being Wellness. This is not a controversial topic, as it is infused in the core of our Western medical paradigm. Where we get stuck in our wellness is when we operate under the belief that physical health is all that matters.

As we walk through the Three Cornerstones of Whole-Being Wellness in the remainder of this book, I am inviting you to dive deeper into who you really are. The purpose of this is to expand your awareness of why the Three Cornerstones of Well-Being are core components of whole-being healing. As you explore these ideas, you may find that you are able to better connect with an appreciation for who you are, and find greater levels of healing yourself.

If this feels like too much for where you are currently in your mental/emotional space, then you can choose to skip over these chapters. If you are game for some fun, I invite you to explore these esoteric topics, which are among my greatest passions.

The first question: We think of ourselves as our physical body, but are we more than that? I invite you now to look a little deeper. To begin, become aware of how we define "me," and by association, how we define our pet. I was first given the opportunity to really evaluate this in the Mahayana Buddhist logic training I embarked upon back in 2004 to help me cope with the significant stressors of my residency and life.

One of the key concepts in those Buddhist esoteric studies was beginning to examine how we define "me," to ask the questions "Who Am I?" and "Where do 'I' begin and end?"

"Who Am I" is also the key question we work with in the ancient metaphysical and hermetic Mystery School lineage in which I am trained and now currently practice. To me, it is interesting to see these age-old questions reflected in ancient world traditions. They exist because they are avenues for us to more accurately understand who we are, who we are not, and how our idea of "me" influences pretty much everything in our life.

Beliefs should be something we hold because we have looked at them from every angle and have proven to OURSELVES that this appears to be true and fits with our current experience. We should not believe something merely because someone told us it is true, or that we are supposed to believe it.

I invite you to consider, just for a moment, what you think of when asked, "Who are you?" It is likely you may think of a number of labels, like your name or your profession. It is also likely that you will conjure up an image of your physical body. So, to a degree, you believe you are your physical body.

But is that true? You have a body, but are you actually your body? See if you can prove that. Okay, so if you are your body, are you your whole body? Or just part of it? You may say, "Of course I am my whole body!" But if that is true, what would happen to "you" if you lost a limb? Would you cease to be you?

You will probably say, "Of course not! I would still be me." Any of us who know a person or maybe a pet who has lost a limb would tell you that the core essence of a person or pet is the same, although the physicality may have changed. So, if you are your body, what part of your body? How much of your body would need to be there for you to still be "you"?

Now, this is a deep conversation and we can't possibly get into the whole thing here in a few short paragraphs. The point I want to make is that sometimes the way we are thinking about things by habit isn't necessarily accurate. I encourage you to start questioning: "Where do 'I' begin and end?"

Why? Because You, the real You, is not simply your physical body – just as your pet is not merely their physical body. How do you know that? Because our physical body can change and the core essence of "us" will still be the same.

So, what is that core essence? We will dive into that as we move forward in this book. While it is very important to care for the physical body, that is not all we are. If we only focus on the physical, we are neglecting essential aspects of "us" – and we will never actually reach true health, balance, wholeness and well-being.

Part II Takeaway

Physical Health

An Approach to Integrative Healing for the Physical Body

Acupuncture
Herbal therapies
Immune support
Gut microbiome health
Select vitamins and supplements
Leveraging whole fresh foods as medicine
Lifestyle factors, exercise and weight management
Limiting exposure to avoidable toxins and carcinogens
Thoughtfully applied Western biomedicine cancer treatments

Focus on Physical Body Health

- Focus on healthy eating, for both yourself and your pet
- Aspire to a healthy weight, limiting caloric intake to what is needed
- Exercise regularly – set a routine for you and your pet to move every day
- Tend to your own health imbalances, as well as your pet's
- Seek to understand and consider all your treatment options

Activity Ideas

- Add one healthy nutritional habit
- Take out one unhealthy nutritional habit
- Switch your pet's treats to healthy ones
- Do one movement activity every day
  - Go for a walk with your dog
  - Run around the house with your cat
  - Do Yoga/Tai Qi or Qi Gong…with your dog or cat in the room
  - Run around the backyard playing catch with your dog
  - Play with your cat to get you both moving
- Give your pet a massage and schedule one for yourself
- Make an appointment to address a lingering health problem of your own
- Tidy up your environment: "As within so without; as without so within."

Esoteric Contemplation Invitation

- Reflect on where "you" begin and where "you" end
- Reflect on where your pet begins and ends. Are they just their physical body?

PART 3

THE SOUL: MIND, EMOTIONS AND ENERGY

Staying Balanced

It is important that, when exploring where you have power to change your behaviors to support well-being, you do not allow yourself to go into guilt, shame or blame. You have lived your life up until now in the best way you knew how and were capable of based on what you knew and the internal resources available to you. Many people have "emotional support" animals exactly because they are stressed, anxious or depressed. Pets help us. And we, in turn, can use that bond to uplift ourselves to greater states with the presence of that support. For example, when we experience emotional support from our companion animals, we can pay attention to what that feels like and work to connect with that feeling in other ways, so we can in turn become a more stable support for them, mutually uplifting each other. Wouldn't it be amazing if the power of the human-animal bond could help motivate us to heal our relationship with ourselves through our desire to, in turn, become the support we would want for them?

Discovering the Missing Puzzle Piece

I have a great driving passion for bringing spirituality to life. You might wonder why that is, given my training as a board-certified veterinary medical oncologist and the significant science training and understanding that requires. Like everyone, I have experienced my own challenges and struggles in life. I experienced extreme burnout at one point, which led me to contemplate abandoning the career that I had spent my entire life building.

In the end, I discovered that my lack of joy and internal sense of fulfillment had nothing to do with my career or external circumstances. It had to do with the fact that I had tried so hard to "fit in" to the world of science and medicine that I had fragmented myself. I had created a huge separation between my spiritual life, which was vivid and real to me, and my physical existence and job, which was acceptable to the world of science and Western medicine in which I had invested so much of my life. That led to what I understand now as a "Soul Sickness," which no amount of medication, supplements, meditation, yoga, exercise, healthy eating or even a career change could fix.

That got worse and eventually led to a critical turning point. I needed help that no one around me was trained to provide. That experience drove me to ask bigger questions and to seek solutions I had previously not been aware existed or willing to believe.

The challenges I have navigated and overcome have given me a lived understanding that allows me to use those learnings to help others. This is the beauty of life and the blessing that exists in every challenge we face. Because of my lived experience and all I have been able to achieve for myself, I know without a doubt that healing, inner peace, strength, emotional balance and physical abundance are possible for everyone who is willing to walk that path of self-discovery and do the work required to create change. The only limits are the ones we place on ourselves, and the blinders we wear keep us from seeing the complete picture of who we are, and what we are truly capable of achieving.

The concepts in this book are applicable to every part of your life. Although here I am using the experience of your pet's cancer to frame this into an actionable series of steps, they can also lead you (if you are willing and open to thinking and living differently) into a field of healing and growth that often is available to us only through the fire of challenge.

The goal, ideally, is to eventually reach a point where we consciously choose growth so that we are able to move forward in our life without the necessity for the "big hits" to push us out of our comfort zone into our next level of awareness.

The reason I have focused my work and life on helping others access the deeper roots of healing and balance, with a specific emphasis on the vital role our Soul and Spirit play in this process, is because I have a heartfelt desire to help others who need and want help, as I did, when I had no idea this kind of help existed.

It isn't that I didn't know that Soul and Spirit were important in our well-being. I grew up in the Christian tradition and had a very real experience of God from a young age. But I didn't have an effective method to mend the disconnect that often happens as we navigate the modern world and all its demands and priorities.

The impact of our mind and emotions and the subtler aspects of our healing are important keys to being able to face life's challenges with greater success. They are also essential to true healing. We are not often supported in accessing these deeper layers of healing.

So much of the focus in the cancer journey is on what we can do to work on a physical level: medicine, surgery, radiation, chemotherapy, food, supplements and physical "alternative medicine" treatments. These are, no doubt, important. But this narrow focus neglects the Soul of who we are, and who our pets are. It doesn't invite us to look deeper into the power of the human-animal bond or acknowledge that we are much more powerful than we are led to believe.

Every experience changes us. Importantly, we participate in HOW those experiences change us. We have a choice in that process. Bringing these aspects into the healing conversation from the start is the best way I know to open the door to living a life that allows us to not merely survive from challenge to challenge, but to make the most of every day.

This book is just a start on opening up the door to that deeper path of healing for you. But it will meet you where you are now, and if you want more, it will connect you with a path forward as far as you choose to go on your journey of healing.

Chapter 9

Stress

There are many things that can cause stress. After a cancer diagnosis in your pet, the most prominent cause of stress for you is likely to arise from what you are thinking and the emotions you are experiencing. This section focuses on a basic understanding of how stress affects you, its impact on well-being, and simple things you can do on your own to alleviate it.

When we have information, we have the opportunity to act on that information in order to effect positive change and better care for ourselves and those in our care. Understanding the impact of stress provides us with a foundation from which to make informed decisions about our habits and take enlightened action toward creating a more optimal experience of life.

By understanding how stress affects you, you can also be more educated about how your stress affects your pet. You can then learn new practices and activities to decrease stress for both of you. Your pet picks up on your "vibes." When you are able to help yourself feel more peaceful, calm and balanced, you will be able to hold that space for your pet as well. Your pet will feel that, and they will want it.

For example, when I meditate at home, my pup Emerald seeks me out and sits on my lap or leans up against me. Being close isn't enough. She likes to be touching me. She loves the calm energy that I am connecting with and embodying during my meditation practice. This is something you can do for your pet too, and it helps you both.

In contrast, Emerald can tell when I am feeling stressed, even if I think I am hiding it pretty well. For example, she rides to work with me, and if we are driving in the car in silence and I start thinking about something that is stressful, she starts whining. Even though I know that pets sense our emotions, it still surprises me, especially since I don't get stressed like I used to. Then I usually laugh and thank her for reminding me to adjust my thoughts and take some deep breaths to connect with calm. When I do that, she settles too.

What Is Stress?

Stress can be understood as your perception of threat and your body's physiological response to it. Stress can affect your mood and emotional responses, leading to anxiety, depression, anger or irritability. Chronic stress results in measurable effects in the physical body, which may contribute to physical illness or disease. Additionally, stress has been shown to decrease cognitive function. In short, stress is a recognized contributing factor to experiencing unhappiness, physical illness and the inability to think clearly.

The physical effects of stress can take a severe toll on your overall well-being and greatly diminish your ability to bounce back after challenging events, or your "resilience." Stress activates the sympathetic nervous system, your "fight, flight or freeze response." Chronic stress can result in the following physical effects:

- Low energy
- Increased cortisol
- Decreased immune function
- Increased Inflammation
- "Cortical inhibition" (stress makes it harder for you to think clearly)
- Premature aging
- Illnesses such as heart disease, inflammatory bowel disease and cancer

The body does not differentiate between "big" stress and "small" stress. Because of this, you can become unaware of the physiological responses to stress you are experiencing, because you get used to chronic stressors and think of your stress as "normal." With enough reinforcement, these stress patterns can become locked into place, making it more and more difficult to return to a state of "neutral," or an unstressed state.

When this kind of unaddressed chronic stress is the baseline, adding a cancer diagnosis in your pet can upset the delicate balance you are maintaining and make just coping with upsetting news feel impossible, not to mention flipping the script to find the opportunities for growth that are present in every challenge.

It is possible, however, with awareness and conscientious behaviors, to manage your stress overload and begin the process of rewiring your habitual stress responses.

Life will always bring ups and downs. That you can't change. But you can control how you interact with these life experiences and how you choose to use them as motivators for developing tools to improve your resilience and overall well-being.

I am not a licensed psychotherapist or counselor. What I am offering in the next two chapters are general practices that are helpful for most people with mild to moderate levels of stress. There are trained therapists that can help you work at the level of your mind to redirect your thoughts and decrease mental and emotional symptoms of more significant stress, anxiety and depression. Depending on the level of stress you are experiencing and other conditions, that kind of professional support may be very helpful for you, at least during this time of challenge.

Your Pet Experiences Your Emotions

Your emotional stress impacts your pet's. I am very interested in the current research in mental and emotional wellness in the human pediatric oncology arena, because there are many parallels to our experiences in veterinary oncology.

We know from human childhood cancer studies that parental distress is associated with long-term distress in pediatric oncology patients. Children whose parents have ongoing chronic stress related to their child's diagnosis exhibit more signs of emotional distress. This illustrates the importance of inter-family dynamics.

Pets are part of the family too, and they experience our emotions. Dogs with cancer are significantly more likely to have shown signs of stress at home prior to diagnosis.[43] This probably isn't surprising to you. Anyone who loves a pet knows that pets pick up on our emotional states. Science has demonstrated this phenomenon.

At least in part, this perception of human emotions seems to be through their strong sense of smell. We transfer emotions to our pets via chemosignals, or chemicals our body produces as a result of different emotions. These have a smell that our dog can detect. Dogs can actually tell the difference between positive and negative emotions and respond differently to different human emotions. When they detect chemosignals associated with anger or fear, they respond differently than they do to those associated with happiness, which has its own smell.[44] Studies have documented that dogs mirror us. They then manifest or experience the emotions corresponding to those their human is experiencing.[45, 46, 47]

Dogs also obtain emotional information from what they see and hear, and integrate it into a coherent perception of human emotion. This means they also pick up on your emotional state through your facial expressions, your body language, your tone of voice and the words themselves.

What does this look like in real life, and how is it relevant to you now?

Imagine this scenario: Bob is worried about his pet, Fluffy, and strongly desires to change her diet to something new. Bob puts the new food in a bowl and offers it to Fluffy. Fluffy smells the new food. Bob stands there anxiously, staring at Fluffy to see if she will eat the food, worried about whether she will accept it. (Prior to the cancer diagnosis, Bob, being a busy guy, used to just put food in the bowl and walk away to his next task.) Fluffy notices this new change in behavior and picks up on stressed emotions from Bob, sensing and then mirroring those emotions. Fluffy feels stressed. Fluffy doesn't eat. Bob feels stressed. Bob doesn't want to eat.

Now imagine this scenario: Bob is excited about the food he is feeding Fluffy and feels good about what he is offering. Bob thinks about how much he loves Fluffy and feels happy he has this moment with her. Bob prepares food with these happy thoughts and feelings. He talks to Fluffy in a happy voice, and explains to her why this food is so good for her and how it is such a big treat she is really going to love. Fluffy watches him prepare this new delicacy while picking up "happy" chemosignals and body language. Bob puts the food in front of Fluffy. Fluffy smells the new food. Bob walks away and goes about his normal behavior. Fluffy feels comfortable with this usual routine. Fluffy eats. Bob feels happy. Fluffy feels happy.

There are many reasons a dog or cat may not want to eat, some of which are medical concerns and some of which may be related to pet preferences. Often, medical tests reveal no obvious cause for reluctance to eat and numerous anti-nausea medications and food changes are not effective at resolving picky eating behaviors. Based on the information above, once we have ruled out a medical cause for poor appetite, we have to also consider how our own emotional state and behavioral changes around feeding time may be affecting our pet. This is just one example of how stress can play a role in the well-being of everyone involved in the care of a pet diagnosed with cancer.

Manage Your Stress to Help Your Pet

All of this research supports the experience that many veterinarians have had in clinical practice. I can't tell you how many times the emotional distress and anxiety of a pet parent during a consultation or veterinary visit visibly affects their pet. It is common to see more anxious behavior in patients whose people are highly anxious. The anxiety exhibited by the pet is often attributed by the pet parent to being at the hospital, not realizing that their emotional state is playing a role in their pet's behavior. The perception of their pet's anxiety often escalates their own, leading to a difficult cycle that makes conversations and veterinary visits even more emotionally and technically challenging for everyone involved.

While there is, undoubtedly, some real stress that many pets experience from the veterinary visit itself, I've had a number of positive results in decreasing anxiety levels when I've had pet parents open to the idea that managing the stress they feel during the visits and at home can help their pet experience less stress. They put effort into learning self-calming techniques and use those at home, on the way to the clinic, and during the visit. For many pets, especially those who are not historically anxious, the positive results can be dramatic.

I am also aware of how my emotional state affects my patients. I try to deliberately enter a room with as much calm as I can muster. I take a few deep breaths before entering, try to think of something positive, and try to be sensitive to the emotional environment of the room when I enter.

When pets are exhibiting signs of fearfulness and anxiety at an initial consultation, for example, if time allows I usually try to sit and talk before approaching them. Many times if I can have a calm exchange with their person, they often settle and show fewer signs of anxiety and fear. Sometimes they even come up to greet me or snuggle when that isn't normal behavior for them at a veterinary visit. My emotions can't often override the emotions of their person, especially if intense, as I believe pets are more acutely attuned to their people than a stranger. But the effort to maintain a calm emotional space can go a long way in improving the experience my patients have during a visit.

This is all just to illustrate that our emotions not only affect us and the humans in our life, but they affect our pets too. This is about understanding. Notice if you are going toward thoughts or feelings of guilt, shame, regret or blame. The point here is not to feel worse about having normal emotions associated with learning your pet has cancer, or to fall into the trap of blaming others. That isn't helpful or effective. The point is to develop an understanding of the dynamics that are at play in our well-being and the well-being of our pets – to learn how we can positively impact each other and support each other while simultaneously supporting our own well-being. When we understand, we have information we can use to make better choices and take positive action.

The good news is that happiness has its own smell, or chemosignals. Happiness, just like negative emotions, can be transferred. So the efforts you make at developing a more genuinely stable emotional landscape and being able to hold happy, peaceful or calm emotional states more often can positively impact your pet during their healing process. If you can learn to "smell happy," your pet might be happier too.

By attending to your own emotional well-being, you will be improving the emotional environment your pet experiences during their veterinary visits and on a daily basis as you share this journey with them. By minimizing your stress, you minimize their stress, which supports their well-being as well as your own. There are many human studies looking at the impact of chronic stress on immune function and healing. We won't get into the details of that here, but will just acknowledge that this is an important consideration if we are looking to support a lifestyle of healing and well-being for yourself and your pet.

A Progressive Relaxation Technique

One of the simplest ways to release stress is by intentionally relaxing the muscles in the body. One of my favorite techniques for this is called "progressive relaxation." Progressive relaxation has been shown to be helpful in reducing cancer caregiver anxiety and to improve the ability to cope with stress.[48] This is something you can do right now, and any time you need to relax or connect with calm. Because of how the body and mind are connected, physical relaxation has a powerful calming influence on the mind.

Try this now:

1. Start by finding a comfortable place to sit or lie down.
2. Allow your attention to settle on your feet and then use the power of your imagination to relax your feet. You can do this by first tensing the muscles in the feet and then relaxing them, or by simply focusing on releasing any muscle tension in the feet. Do this three times.
3. Then move up your body, repeating the same process with each part of the body until you reach the top of your head. For example: lower legs, knees, upper legs, hips and pelvis, lower back, upper back, chest, hands, arms, shoulders, neck, jaw, face, eyes, forehead and scalp.
4. Then simply rest, enjoying the relaxation you have created in the body.

You can do this with your pet resting in your lap or nearby. Notice if they seem to respond to your relaxation too. They might also find it relaxing.

Other Ways to Alleviate Stress

Take a deep breath: Your breath is always available to you everywhere you go, and it's free. Deep breathing is proven to calm the nervous system and shift you from a state of stress ("fight or flight" sympathetic nervous system response) to a state of greater calm, allowing the parasympathetic nervous system (the "rest and digest" side of your nervous system) to engage. You can do these breathing exercises anywhere: at home, in the car, even at the grocery store if your mind starts wandering to stressful events. You can also do this with your pet on the way to the veterinary hospital, or before it is time to give them their medications. You set the tone and they will take your lead. You can even put your hand on your pet's chest as you breathe, and notice whether their breathing seems to calm too.

Simple 4 Count Breathing Exercise:

1. Allow your attention to focus on the sensations of the breath, wherever you notice them most strongly. This might be at the nostrils where the air moves in and out; cooler on the inhale, warmer on the exhale. Or it might be in the rising and falling of the chest or belly.
2. Simply notice the breath for a few moments without trying to change it.

3. Now, begin to lengthen the breaths to a comfortable level according to your own pacing. You never want to become short of breath. You simply want to take deeper, slower breaths than usual.
4. Now, to the pace that is comfortable for you, count to four on the inhale and then count to four on the exhale.
5. Optional: If you are feeling anxious, you may choose to gently pause at the bottom of the exhale for a moment, before you inhale. If you are feeling tired or depressed, you may choose to gently pause at the top of the inhale for a moment before the exhale.
6. Continue this pattern, in a relaxed way, for 11 rounds. Or set a timer to do this for a few minutes so you can relax your mind and allow the timer to cue you when you are finished.

Walk outside in nature: Forest bathing has been getting more and more attention as a beneficial activity to decrease stress. The beauty of nature is calming. But getting out among the trees can have even more benefits.[49, 50] Take a walk with your dog. If you can do this with your kitty without causing stress in the transition, consider getting a safe place for your kitty to enjoy the outdoors with you, or a kitty harness, so you can both breathe the fresh air. There are pet strollers now that are zipped up to keep your pets from jumping out. This could be a fun activity for you if you both enjoy it.

Professional help: Taking care of your emotional self is extremely important. It can be very helpful to seek professional help when you are experiencing intense emotions that have become challenging for you to manage. Many people neglect to seek out help due to a fear of appearing weak, fragile or "broken." In fact, taking steps to seek the help you need is a great sign of strength. It is also the most compassionate thing you can do for yourself, your pet and everyone else in your life. We all need a little help once in a while. Fortunately, there are people who have dedicated their life to helping us find balance during challenging times.

When we address stress from multiple angles and utilize all the resources at our disposal, we can optimize results. It is also important to know that you are not alone on this journey and that you can be empowered to create a more peaceful emotional foundation.

CHAPTER 9 CHECK-IN

- Sit with your pet on your lap and gently place your hand on them or massage them, connecting in a calm way. Then do one of the stress-relieving activities from this chapter and see if they seem to enjoy it:
    - Progressive relaxation technique
    - Simple 4 Count Breathing
- Go for a walk in nature and breathe in the fresh air. If you can find a place with trees, even better! Bring your dog with you on your walk if they can go on a walk with you. They will enjoy it too.
- Bring some trees or cat-safe plants into your home. This will bring a little nature indoors.

Chapter 10

Calming the Mind

Since the beginning of time, spiritual traditions have supported humans with practices designed to help us navigate life more successfully. These practices demonstrate a deep understanding of how the human mind and emotions work. It is fascinating to read modern scientific research, which is being used to validate what ancient traditions have known for thousands of years. These ancient practices have stood the test of time precisely *because* they work. They help us.

In the modern age, the scientific method has become the standard by which we measure the effectiveness or validity of any kind of intervention. This is a valuable approach to providing information we can use to guide our lifestyle and healing choices. While this approach is limited by our current level of understanding and ability to measure various phenomena of the human structure, it has proven valuable in assisting some of these ancient practices in making their way into the modern medicine paradigm. As we continue to evolve as a species and our understanding grows, we will be able to gain greater and greater insights that will continue to progress our approach to health and healing.

There are many exciting advancements happening all the time. Again, that is not the focus of this book. But I do want to expand on some ancient spiritual practices that have been incorporated into many mental health approaches and are becoming more "mainstream."

Improving your ability to remain calm and centered helps your pet.

When you are feeling more balanced and centered, you will feel better. This will make it easier for you to stay focused on what is important and appreciate every day. You will have more capacity to take care of your pet, who will likely require a much more expanded care routine than they used to, and to do so with some feelings of peace that you are doing something good for them. They will be the happy beneficiary of your better mood, and their quality of life will improve too because they will feel you are more at ease. Remember, you are the center of their universe.

Any of the practices below can become quality time with your pet by including them in your practice. They can sit with you as you do the practices and connect with calm. You can also use your gratitude and love for them as a focus of a mindfulness practice, for example.

Mindfulness

Increased mindfulness, awareness and attention to the present moment, significantly decreases symptoms of depression and anxiety in cancer patient caregivers.[51] It has been shown to significantly decrease distress, stress and negative thoughts, and to increase the ability to experience positive personal growth through the cancer patient caregiving journey.[52]

Mindfulness Practices to Reduce Stress

Mindfulness-like practices can be traced back to Vedic and pre-Buddhist India as early as 1500 BCE. The Upanishads (c. 800–500 BCE), spiritual texts that encourage self-reflection and the discovery of who we are underneath our everyday life, explore things like self-inquiry, stillness and inner realization. These ideas helped shape the contemplative traditions of Buddhism, where meditation was more formally developed as a practice. Similar themes of inner awareness and stillness appear across other spiritual traditions, including contemplative Christian movements and modern spirituality.

Mindfulness is now commonly talked about in mental health circles, so I want to share some of my experience and the research around this here. While it can be very helpful for many people, it isn't for everyone because there are some significant considerations for those who are in the midst of a crisis or trauma. However, it may be a useful tool for you to add to your toolbox.

The Benefits of Mindfulness Practices

Mindfulness is defined as a state of active, open attention that focuses on observing what is happening right now, in the present moment, without judging it. Mindfulness helps you stay aware of what is happening now, rather than dwelling on the past or anticipating the future.

Mindfulness practices have been around for eons and are used in modern psychotherapy to alleviate anxiety, depression and other mood imbalances. A lot of research has been published on how these ancient and modern mindfulness practices work on the brain and mood states.

Mindfulness stress reduction practices may be beneficial in the following ways:

1. Mitigating anxiety, depression and emotional extremes
2. Developing resilience
3. Appreciating the present moment
4. Improving physical well-being
5. Accepting and supporting yourself and others in healthy ways

Enhanced awareness and attention regulation – as well as acceptance of thoughts, emotions and states without feeling the need to invest in, alter or escape from them – are just a few of the benefits experienced as a result of mindfulness practices.[53] Regular mindfulness practice has been shown to improve prosocial behaviors, benefiting not only yourself but others around you.[54] It results in increased ability for emotional acceptance and results in "cortical facilitation" – that is, it promotes clear thinking. Regular mindfulness practice is proven to improve symptoms of burnout, stress, anxiety and depression in health care workers.[55]

There is a growing body of evidence demonstrating the benefit of Mindfulness-Based Stress Reduction (MBSR). Short-term training programs have demonstrated measurable improvement in cancer caregiver quality of life, decreased caregiver burden, and improved readiness to engage in treatment planning.[56]

The Limitations of Mindfulness

While mindfulness has an important place in becoming more self-aware, its use has limitations. Most notably, bringing more awareness to challenging emotional states can potentially increase anxiety or mental-emotional stress. It is important to be aware of this as you are navigating your cancer care journey, and life in general. If at any point you feel that a practice or technique is not helping you, be gentle with yourself and seek professional support. In addition, mindfulness requires effort and a willingness to do something to help yourself. Some people are not in a place they can or want to do that, so other methods may be more appropriate until you get to the point that you are able and willing to help yourself move forward.

While there are potential adverse effects from almost every intervention because we are all individuals, it is also important to keep things in perspective. For example, a randomized clinical trial performed in 2023 evaluated results between two groups.

One group received an antidepressant pharmaceutical drug, and the other received eight sessions of weekly Mindfulness-Based Stress Reduction (MBSR) training. The study showed the two interventions to be of equal effectiveness. Interestingly, treatment-related adverse events occurred in 78.6% of patients in the pharmaceutical intervention group but only 15.4% of patients in the MBSR group. This difference was statistically significant. While a variety of physical side effects were reported in the pharmaceutical intervention group, the only adverse event in the MBSR group was increased anxiety.[57]

Practically speaking, mindfulness can help you become more aware of your thoughts and how they are affecting you. This is beneficial because you need to be aware of something before you can change it. Mindfulness, then, is a tool you can use to become aware of your internal dialogue so that you can assess, with kindness and without judging, where it may be helpful to make adjustments.

Then you must choose to take action to adjust. Because being aware of a situation doesn't change the underlying dynamic that has created the situation, it is important to understand that the mindfulness practice itself does not solve the problem of where troubling thoughts are coming from. It does, however, help you to accept they are there from an observer's perspective instead of identifying with them.

As you observe your thoughts, you can create some space to realize you are not actually your thoughts. You are *experiencing* thoughts. From there you can choose to engage with them at a different level. You can choose to pause before acting and then to decide how you want to engage with that thought as you move forward.

In that sense, mindfulness is not the ultimate be-all and end-all. It's a helpful tool you can use to accept and become more aware. In any self-mastery endeavor, this is a crucial skill. Then you will need to engage other methods or healings to make the adjustments to address the root cause of those thoughts. Before you have other tools (you can learn them with me or with anyone else you wish to study with who resonates with your interests and goals), mindfulness itself will still be helpful because while it doesn't get rid of negative thoughts, it significantly reduces their power over you.

Learning Mindfulness

You don't need to commit to an hour a day in order to benefit from mindfulness practices. Mindfulness practices are a way to create new habits in your mind that support your well-being and overall effectiveness in life. Many simple practices that can be done in 5–15 minutes will reap tangible benefits in your life. With practice and consistency, you will learn to LIVE mindfully, engaging in mindful awareness throughout your day – not just when you are sitting quietly at home.

While you can't control whether most of the events you experience in life happen, you can learn methods to navigate those experiences with more ease and grace.

With practice, those new habits become second nature, and you will soon find that things that used to feel difficult no longer feel quite so challenging. You are better able to access uplifted feelings. You become calmer. When you are more calm and peaceful, that positively impacts everything you do. You are able to offer more to those you care about. You are able to be a better caregiver, parent, spouse, sibling, friend and community member.

Giving yourself the tools to find balance amidst the chaos and challenges of life is one of the best gifts you can give yourself and everyone around you, including your pet.

The Present Moment

One of the things we can learn from our pets is the power of staying in the present moment. Pets are good at living in the moment. Most of the time our human mind is caught up in the past or the future. When we send our mind into the past we can get caught up in blame, guilt or regret. We have no power to change the past. Our power is in the present moment, in the choices we make right now. When we send our mind into the future, we can get trapped in worry or anxiety, as we often worry about things that may not ever happen. Fear of the unknown, of what the future might bring, steals the moments you have now. Mindfulness practices train us to bring our attention to what is happening right now. When we allow our attention to settle in this present moment, there is a deep relaxing that can happen.

Breathing, Senses and Sound

Breathing

Deep, slow, deliberate breathing short-circuits the "fight or flight" stress response and engages the parasympathetic nervous system. It has been proposed that, compared to neurotransmitter-targeting medications, self-regulated breathing may more effectively address the whole-body imbalances that occur in stress, anxiety and depression. Certain types of meditation, relaxation and breathing techniques have been shown to mitigate the detrimental effects of negative emotional states and the sympathetic dominance of the autonomic nervous system associated with chronic stress and anxiety.[58]

Sensory Absorption

This is a practice of focusing your awareness on the sensory experiences at hand. In this process, you work toward fully enjoying a sensory experience. This refocuses the mind from thoughts of the past and future to what is happening right now in the present moment. This practice can engage any of the senses: smell, touch, sight, taste or hearing. The goal is to experience a feeling of enjoyment while becoming immersed in the sensation.

Sound

Mantra is a healing practice that has been in use for centuries. Modern research into the physiological effects of mantra showed beneficial brain changes on functional MRI with "om" chanting compared to control groups who made "ssss" sounds or rested quietly. These changes were noted in certain areas of the brain: the amygdala, anterior cingulate gyrus, hippocampus, insula, orbitofrontal cortex, parahippocampal gyrus and thalamus regions. These effects seemed to be primarily due to vagal nerve activation through the branches associated with hearing. Vagal nerve activation is one method used to treat depression due to its ability to calm overactive areas of the brain associated with depression.[59]

Classical music can alleviate stress and also has a calming effect in dogs.[60]

Meditation

There are many other types of meditation you can explore to help you with stress management, calming the thoughts, releasing emotions, and generally experiencing more calm. Most of them do not have published research on their application in the cancer caregiver setting. I have focused on mindfulness here because it has garnered a lot of attention in the medical community, so have research studies that have been published. Loving Kindness Meditation is another type of meditation that has received a lot of attention. It is one of the most researched meditation methods, although it has comparatively fewer published research articles directly pertaining to the cancer caregiver setting. The studies that have been published show that regular Loving Kindness Meditation can improve measures of stress, self-compassion, social connectedness, resilience, hope and quality of life in people on the cancer caregiver journey.[61, 62]

I have taught many types of meditation over the years: Loving Kindness Meditation (traditionally called Metta Meditation), mindfulness practices logic and contemplative meditations in the Mahayana Buddhist tradition, as well as inner body meditations, which focus on visualization of the energies in the body. I have found that a major obstacle for most people new to meditation practice is racing thoughts and a busy mind. For many people this is frustrating enough to cause them to abandon meditation altogether and to claim it is "impossible" for them to meditate.

As part of my training in the Mystery School tradition, I learned to guide a meditation technique called Max Meditation System™. This meditation technique combines ancient yogic traditions, modern psychology and neuro-linguistic programming. In my experience teaching meditation, this has been the most effective meditation technique to help people access states of stillness quickly. I often have students attend Max Meditation System™ events who say, "I can't meditate. I've tried but my mind is so busy I can't calm it down." It is rewarding to see how many of them are smiling and calm by the end of their first session, having experienced a still mind for the very first time. It gives them the experience of success, which gives them hope and shifts their belief from "I can't" to "I can." As of the time of this writing, I teach this meditation monthly to support those who are interested in alleviating stress and calming their busy mind.

The Power of Consistency

A major limitation to the effectiveness of meditation practices is consistency and follow-through. Studies show that to experience the best results, these practices need to be done regularly over time. Many of the published studies I have cited show that only about one-third of the participants engaged with the practices regularly, and these were the people who experienced results.

This tells us that the willingness to create new self-care habits, or lifestyle changes, is imperative if you want to experience greater well-being. That might seem obvious, but it is very common for people to give up on a new practice before it has even had adequate time to have a notable effect. Meditation can and does have immediate benefits, but for these to last long beyond the relaxation of the meditation session itself, regularity is needed.

This is because in order for us to experience ourselves and our lives differently, we have to DO our life differently. We have to learn how to BE in our life in a different way. This is one of the limits of relying on willpower, which is often lacking during stressful times. It's the main reason I have found that other interventions that provide deeper levels of energetic support and healing, which I speak about as we go further in the book, can be pivotal to supporting people in making the internal shifts necessary to *desire* to take care of themselves and to uplevel their lifestyle to support higher levels of wellness. The mind only gets us so far.

The Limits of the Mind

While the mind is powerful, and needs to be trained, there are limits to what the mind alone can do. I know from personal experience. My oncology residency training program was extremely stressful and was significantly affecting my quality of life. My mind was busy and going into a lot of negative stories, and I was exhausted. I knew this wasn't healthy for me.

Thankfully, I knew enough to know there was a better way to live. That inner nudge led me to seek out yoga as a way of managing stress. Yoga led me to explore meditation. That connected me with a way to deeply study the workings of the mind and a concrete method of mind training. Putting what I learned into practice, I experienced the power of the mind to manage stress responses and help me step out of limiting beliefs. I also experienced its limits.

All that mind training brought me to a threshold that I couldn't get past despite all the things I had learned and knew. When you get too focused on mental processes, you get stuck at the level of your thoughts, which are really just reflections of, or symptoms of, the deeper conditions or patterns underneath. Without addressing the root cause of your thoughts and emotions, you enter a never-ending battle of subduing, redirecting and reframing them as the same patterns continue to reassert themselves over and over.

I did get very good at controlling my thoughts and not giving them as much power over my choices and actions. And that served me well. It did help me to be less disturbed by the things that were going on around me. It definitely helped me cope better with the stressors of my residency training and clinical practice. But the constant mental chatter was always there, running in the background.

I share this because I know most of you reading this book have that chatty inner voice too. I know that because when I mention this to clients and those who come to study metaphysical spirituality with me, almost everyone nods and laughs. Many often relate animated stories of how their thoughts regularly cause them trouble. We often get a good laugh when I ask, "How many of you can't sleep at night because you are lying awake thinking about all the amazing things that are happening?" We laugh because we all experience that it isn't the good thoughts that cause us trouble. It's the negative ones. Keeping that negative voice at bay takes a certain amount of energy and attention. And it can be exhausting.

When you are immersed in the stress and worry that often accompanies cancer patient caregiving, this can amplify the upsetting thoughts that you are experiencing. Additionally, one of the things that leads to an even busier mind is low energy or exhaustion. Intense emotions can steal your energy, making it even more challenging to find the inner stillness and quiet you will crave during this time. Believe me when I tell you I understand what you are probably experiencing now and the trouble that inner voice can bring you. I'm here to tell you there is hope. There is always more for those who want it. Even in the midst of challenging life events, the mind *can* become quiet, the inner voice calm.

How? The only way I know to do that effectively is the path that I walked to get here. It requires an integrative approach, taking all this mind work deeper into the realms of energy, Spirit and potential. If you want to know more, continue with me on this journey and I will walk you through the process of opening up to the possibilities.

Your mind is powerful. While positive thinking isn't enough to cure cancer or to permanently eliminate all your troubles, learning to master your thoughts and emotions is an essential component to achieving well-being and experiencing inner peace. Understanding your thoughts and emotions and the role they play, where they come from, and how to heal so that you are more in balance is a journey beyond the scope of this book. That journey is a way of living, healing and creating balance inside of you.

That isn't something you can learn from reading a book. It is something you become through lived experience and a conscious decision to let go of your old coping mechanisms and the belief systems that are keeping you stuck in cycles of suffering. It is something that comes about by choosing to BE in your life in a new way. This is the journey I facilitate in my healing center for humans. But you can begin the first steps of that journey now.

The first step is becoming aware and taking small steps toward calming your mental chatter and relaxing every day so that you can allow yourself to enjoy the moments you have.

The next step is energy.

CHAPTER 10 CHECK-IN

Choose one or more practices to do three times a week or more.

Mindfulness:

- Attend a local center for a guided mindfulness meditation practice.
- Download one of the many mindfulness apps available now and listen to one meditation every day or three times per week.
- If you have trouble connecting with a local instructor, many books have been published on mindfulness practices, which can be purchased at any bookseller. Many of these books are written for people with no previous experience and are very accessible.
- Simply sit and watch the thoughts arising in your mind. Practice imagining that each thought is like a cloud floating through your mind and simply watch the thought clouds float by without following them. This helps you learn not to get wrapped up in every thought going through your head.
- A water fountain in the house can be a nice touch to create a calming ambiance and act as a nice focal point for you to sit and enjoy the sound of the moving water.

Gratitude:

- Write in a journal three things you are grateful for each night before you go to bed, or each morning before you start the day.

Sensory Absorption:

- Put on some relaxing classical music and sit with your pet and relax, really listening to all the details of the music.
- Spend some time gently massaging your pet and really allow yourself to pay attention to what you are feeling – the sensations of their fur on your hand, for example, and how it feels different in different areas.
- Play a game with your pet and really immerse yourself in the moment. Allow yourself to enjoy and laugh.
- Go on a walk with your dog and get out of your head and into your senses. Really focus on the things you see and the sounds you hear. How does the ground feel beneath your feet? Can you smell the trees?

Meditation:

- Find a local meditation group.
- I teach meditation regularly. You may not be local to me, but there may be a local meditation group in your area with which you can participate and meet a community of supportive friends. In-person experiences bring another level of benefit to meditation.
- Explore online guided meditation options.

- I have a number of guided meditations and may currently be offering free guided meditation sessions on my website. You can check out my offerings in the Appendix.
- Many other people provide guided online meditations as well. Find someone you resonate with and a practice you will stick with.
- The best meditation practice is the one you will actually DO.

A real-life example of incorporating meditation into your pet's care:

One of my clients, Rachel, shared with me a favorite memory. Every morning, first thing when she got up, she would give Buddy one of his supplements that had to be given on an empty stomach at least 20–30 minutes before breakfast. They would then go snuggle in bed while they listened to one of my recorded meditations together for 20 minutes before breakfast. She shared that she was mostly doing it for him, as she would not have done it for just herself. But for her it was a beautiful time together and a really special way to begin every day. And it helped her.

So you might do something like this with your little furry loved one. You might be surprised by how much it helps you both.

Energy is not an alternative to biology. It is another lens through which we can understand the living system. The future of healing will not come from abandoning science, nor from mistaking its current edge as the limits of reality, but from continually expanding our understanding of what it means to be alive.

Chapter 11

The Energy Body

At the core, we are all energy. Energy healing has been a foundational aspect of traditional healing systems for millennia. Energy healing works with the energy field of the body, also called the biofield. One of the main ways energy healing has historically been applied is through hands-on healing. We can appreciate the innate nature of this healing by just observing our own behavior when we become injured. What is the first thing you do when you cut yourself or sustain an injury? You put your hands over it. This isn't by accident. It is instinctual for a reason. And while you might argue that putting your hands over a broken bone won't set and heal it, you cannot realistically argue that it doesn't help alleviate some of the pain or have any other beneficial effect.

There is an energy emitted by the hands. You can experiment with this yourself by doing a simple exercise that I was reminded of by one of my mentors in the Modern Mystery School, Ipsissima Dr. Theresa Bullard. First, clap your hands and then rub your palms together rapidly for 30–60 seconds, until you feel heat between your palms. Then slowly start to glide your hands past each other without them touching. Notice what you feel. You may also hold your hands out in front of you, about one foot apart with palms facing each other, like holding a ball. Become still and calm and pay attention to the sensation at your palms, breathing deeply. As you do this, slowly move your hands toward each other until they are almost touching. When does the sensation on your palms change? What do you sense? Slowly move your hands further apart and closer together as you pay attention to any gradient in the energy, shifts in pressure, or a sensation like magnets attracting and repelling.

The biofield is a documented phenomenon, and research on the influence of the biofield in health and healing is gaining interest in the Western world. However, inconsistent documentation as well as cultural, institutional and belief system obstacles have limited the research on these therapies for specific conditions. While these limitations may have affected the generalized acceptance and integration of these interventions into conventional Western medicine mindset and training, there is growing interest by patients, practitioners and researchers who have witnessed and personally experienced the beneficial effects firsthand. At the time of this publication, Reiki, a form of hands-on energy healing, is being offered in a growing number of hospital systems in the United States, including prestigious hospitals such as MD Anderson, Memorial Sloan Kettering Cancer Center, and Johns Hopkins Hospital and Health Centers.[63]

While the many biofield therapies have not made their way solidly into the U.S. general mainstream Western medical system yet, we have been using energy medicine for a long time.

We tend to have a greater acceptance of things we can see with the naked eye, or measure with our current instrumentation. If you need to start with things that feel more concrete and tangible, radiation therapy – which aims a beam of invisible energy at a tumor – is a type of energy medicine.

Radiation therapy, though invisible itself, results in visible damage and pain to normal tissues, so it is not possible to convince ourselves that it is imaginary. We can also document tumor shrinkage with many radiation modalities. As our technology is improving, we have developed radiation modalities that are able to target and deliver more energy directly to the tumor tissue so that there are fewer side effects to normal tissues.

Laser therapy is another example of energy medicine. It is backed by research and used in the treatment of a number of physical ailments to aid in tissue repair. It has even been used to aid healing of radiation side effects and to promote tissue healing in nonhealing wounds occurring after cancer surgery.[64, 65] Lasers have been used for surgical techniques and to treat cancer.[66, 67]

These high-intensity energy treatments are primarily aimed to work on the physical body level. What if there were a way to work on the more subtle aspects of the biofield? Might there be a way to address the energetic scaffolding of the body in a way that would support healing? It seems possible, based on research articles showing that Reiki healing resulted in measurable improvement in the immune system of cancer patients.

Reiki

Biofield healing modalities like Reiki have been in use for centuries, and in the past few decades they have gained wider acceptance even in the Western medical system. Reiki has been shown to help alleviate stress in cancer patient caregivers.[68] Reiki treatments have also shown benefit in decreasing pain, anxiety and stress in human cancer patients and have been shown to generally improve quality of life.[69, 70, 71, 72, 73] In animal experiments, Biofield therapy has been shown to positively affect the immune system in cancer-bearing mice.[74, 75]

While research suggests quality of life benefits for both cancer patients and caregivers, to date there are not adequate studies evaluating Reiki's role in tumor control. And while there is some research showing that Reiki might provide beneficial alterations in tumor micro-environment and the immune system, the number of research studies looking into these effects is sparse. Until someone takes up the mantle to do more research in this area, there will be unanswered questions as to the full role energy healing modalities like Reiki and other types of energy healing modalities might play in cancer patient care, beyond the ability to alleviate emotional imbalance or support the immune system.

Research into new fields of treatment and patient care is time-consuming and expensive. It also typically takes 20–40 years for published data to shift the current paradigm, incorporating new practices into the Western medical system and adopting them into what is considered "standard of care." Personal experience and a long tradition of use have allowed this safe, basic human biofield healing instinct to endure and aid many people and animals.

Now that we have addressed what we do and don't know about the science and current state of the research, I would like to share my personal experience and offer for your consideration some practices you might explore to support you and your pet during this challenging time.

It is not my goal to make claims about efficacy or guarantee results – only to make you aware of healing modalities that may support you in your cancer patient care journey, and which I have seen help many who have chosen to explore them with a qualified practitioner. You can decide for yourself whether you feel these approaches are interesting or beneficial to you.

Addressing healing at the energetic level can be a powerful way to support physical, mental and emotional health and healing. While we are gaining a greater understanding of the mechanisms of action of energy medicine and the beneficial effects of energy medicine modalities, there is still a lot we can't explain with the popular science we currently use to explain our universe. Yet the results experienced by those receiving this type of healing support should, even if you are not inclined to believe its validity, at least cause an intelligent and curious mind to entertain there is more to it than just imagination.

Pets, for example, do not experience the placebo effect in the same way people do. When they respond with increased energy, improved appetite or even decreased pain, this cannot rationally be attributed to wishful thinking. Pets don't think and imagine in the same way humans do.

Despite the apparent lack of interest in running clinical trials on the effects of Reiki on tumor progression based on the paucity of published research studies, Reiki practitioners like myself have personal stories of interesting tumor remissions and unexpected survival benefits in cancer patients who receive Reiki as part of their cancer therapy. The fact remains that adverse effects from Reiki therapy are extremely rare, and there is at least repeatedly demonstrated psycho-emotional benefit. So it makes sense to consider this as a part of whole-being patient-centered cancer care.

I have been trained in Reiki since 2003. My current preferred technique is a type of Reiki called Ensofic Reiki™. I have performed Ensofic Ray Reiki™ for many veterinary patients and human clients alike. The animals I have treated with this modality do seem to enjoy it, and clients often report improvement in their pet's demeanor and vitality as well as their own. Pets receive this treatment readily and almost always become very relaxed and at ease. This can be a very helpful option to decrease anxiousness in both people and pets. It also may help alleviate symptoms of cancer. The most common comment I receive from clients after receiving an Ensofic Ray Reiki™ session is that they feel more peaceful and relaxed. And pets often show improved energy levels.

I would never promise specific results, but in my experience this is a powerful option to add to a comprehensive cancer patient care protocol. I have personal experience with friends who have received regular Ensofic Ray Reiki™ sessions while they are receiving chemotherapy treatments, and they often share that their medical care team comments on how well they are handling treatments. Pets are no different, although they cannot express their experiences in the same way a person can. I even know humans who are exceeding their expected survival time when incorporating regular Ensofic Ray Reiki™ sessions into their weekly protocols.

Like every treatment, some patients respond differently than others and I cannot guarantee specific results for your pet. Nevertheless, energy healing modalities are worth considering as part of a comprehensive treatment approach to optimize outcomes if you are interested in working at this level as part of the three cornerstones (Body/Soul/Spirit) approach to wellness and healing. In my experience, they can be a powerful way to support well-being and healing, adding another dimension to the other healing modalities you are pursuing.

The biggest challenge in accurately assessing the full potential of these treatments is client follow-through. There are few clients who have been motivated enough to pursue weekly Ensofic Ray Reiki™ sessions for their pet. This is usually a combination of skepticism, overwhelm and financial concerns. However, I often wonder what we might achieve with regular sessions in our veterinary cancer patient care, given what I have seen in humans – especially since distance healing sessions are so easy to deliver to pets in the comfort of their own home.

In addition to Ensofic Rey Reiki™, I also practice a number of energy and metaphysical healing modalities. The best single energy intervention I have seen help release stress and work at multiple levels is a metaphysical healing modality called Life Activation. (If you are curious to learn more about Life Activation or other healing modalities I offer, please see the Appendix.)

Revisiting Acupuncture

One of the things I appreciate about the Chinese medicine paradigm is the way it acknowledges the interconnection of the various dimensions of our well-being and health – physical, mental, emotional and spiritual. Energy is at the core of health and healing in many ancient traditions. The vital life force that runs through us is, in these ancient traditions, a primary focus of healing interventions. Each tradition had its own name for this vital life force. It is known as Qi, pronounced "chi," in Chinese medicine. Other names are *Prana* in Yogic and Ayurvedic traditions and *Lung*, pronounced "loong," in Tibetan traditions. When that vital life force is out of balance, weak, blocked or not circulating properly, it is understood that various imbalances occur that can manifest at any number of different levels: mental, emotional, physical and spiritual. In this way, it is understood that healthy and proper flow of energy is necessary for health and optimal well-being, and that all disease can ultimately be traced to disturbances in that energy, or vital life force.

As a very simple example, in Chinese medicine the Liver is seen as a physical organ, like modern medicine. It can be affected by disease itself. But it is also an important member of the orchestra of the entire body. Imbalances in the liver are recognized to cause problems distant from the physical liver itself.

Unlike modern Western medicine, in Chinese medicine each organ has an associated emotion and an aspect or expression of Spirit. The emotion or Spirit can be out of balance even if the physical organ itself is still performing its physiological functions. For the liver, for example, the emotion is anger. When the energy flow of the liver is disrupted, it can manifest as frustration or resentment. The spirit of the liver is called the *Hun* and is related to our ability to bring our dreams to fruition. In this way we can see that a more holistic view of balance, health and healing exists in which the interplay of the physical, emotional and spiritual aspects of our existence is woven together.

In Chinese medicine there are five aspects of "Spirit" (in the Chinese medicine definition of the term) that support the Soul. Each is associated with an organ and an emotion.[76] It is important to remember that emotions are normal. Emotions are unbalanced when they become excessive or unrelenting. This is interesting to contemplate because there are actions one can take to help move through imbalanced emotional states. Are you experiencing any of these?

Heart:

- Spirit: Shen: Mind – All feeling and overarching consciousness
- Positive expression: Joy
- Emotion when out of balance: Guilt or shame
- Expression when out of balance: Low self-esteem, paranoia, erratic behavior, disordered thoughts, excessive attachment
- Activity: Connect in positive ways with others in a healthy relationship

Lungs:

- Spirit: Po: Corporeal Soul
- Positive expression: Healthy sense of individuality, resilience
- Emotion when out of balance: Grief
- Expression when out of balance: Lack of vigor and vitality
- Activity: Staying connected to the present moment through breathing

Liver:

- Spirit: Hun: Ethereal Soul
- Positive Expression: Courage, effective planning, able to face difficulties
- Emotion when out of balance: Anger, resentment or timidity
- Expression when out of balance: Lack of direction and inspiration in life

- Activity: Pursuit of goals and dreams and planning what is needed to accomplish them

Spleen:

- Spirit: Yi: Intellect
- Positive expression: Clear thinking, concentration, generating ideas
- Emotion when out of balance: Worry or overthinking
- Expression when out of balance: Sluggish thinking, difficulty focusing
- Activity: Establish clear goals and engage actively with focused attention

Kidneys:

- Spirit: Zhi: Willpower
- Positive expression: Memory, determination and drive to pursue goals
- Emotion when out of balance: Fear
- Expression when out of balance: Desire to run away from your life
- Activity: Ask "What do I want? What am I waiting for?"

This is just one way to conceptualize the interweaving of Mind, Emotion and Spirit into every facet of our life. But it is one of the things I value about Chinese medicine. There are links between the physical, the Soul (mental/emotional) and the Spirit. Do you have any physical ailments that are also expressed as the associated emotion listed above? It's interesting to think about the interconnection. You might consider playing with the suggested activity above to see if you notice any changes – or even working with a licensed Chinese medicine practitioner.

While it is important to treat the physical, treating the Soul and Spirit is just as important to healing. During my decades of practice, I have personally experienced both the benefits and the limitations of conventional Western medicine, herbal medicine, acupuncture, diet, meditation, psychotherapy and various energy medicine treatment modalities. What has fascinated me the most on my journey to find better answers are the dramatic shifts that can occur when working on a metaphysical level with ancient healing modalities, which have been preserved through the centuries. These modalities reach into what you could understand as the quantum realm, the field of potential. They are called "metaphysical" because they work beyond the physical. The Soul, with its mental and emotional component, is still part physical. These metaphysical modalities are spiritual healing modalities. I usually describe them as working on the level of your spiritual blueprint – the foundational imprint and sacred geometry that is "You," in the larger sense.

In PART IV, we are going to expand on this last component of our wellness, spiritual health, and what that practically means in our journey of life, healing and well-being.

CHAPTER 11 CHECK-IN

There is a nonvisible part of our body that science calls the biofield. It is possible to work directly with the biofield to support well-being.

In the Eastern healing traditions, emotions and the energetic state of the body have been recognized as important in health and healing for centuries and longer. Energy healing modalities like Reiki are now being offered in many hospital settings and integrative oncology centers for humans.

Alternative Healing Support

Energy Healing: Reiki or Ensofic Ray Reiki™

- This can be done for pets and humans, both in person or remotely.
- People have shared they have experienced the following potential benefits:
  - Physical support: Strengthened immune system, assisting healing processes, and relieving physical tension or imbalance
  - Mental and emotional clearing: Releasing unhelpful patterns, attachments and stress responses
  - Deep peace and reset: Improved calm, centeredness and clarity

    - Flexible and accessible: Receive healing from anywhere – especially supportive during illness, recovery or times of emotional strain

Metaphysical Healing: Life Activation Session

- People receiving this ancient energy activation have shared that they experienced the following potential benefits:
    - Greater mental clarity: Clear confusion and make decisions with more confidence.
    - Reduced stress and anxiety: Calm your mind and nervous system for greater inner peace.
    - Moving through stagnation and apathy: Release limiting thoughts and step into new possibilities, hope and acceptance.
    - Improved passion and sense of purpose: Feel more connected to yourself with greater meaning and purpose in life.
    - Increased energy and motivation: Feel recharged and supported to take more aligned action to help yourself and your pet.
- The last part of this session can also be done for pets.
    - This may help improve healing.
    - Commonly, pets feel calmer and may have improved energy.

Chapter 12

Diving Deeper: Soul Purpose

As I invite you deeper into the topic of Soul, I want to share a beautiful and powerful story of how our animal companions can act as guides for us, opening us up to greater possibility and even connecting us with our Soul Purpose and life mission. This is my dear friend Ashley White's story in her own words. She is a Guide in the lineage of King Salomon, like I am. This is the story of how her incredible bond with her cat set her on a course that connected her with her Soul Purpose.

Death is a catalyst to change.

Yet it's hardly ever an easy process – especially when it's your furry friend who has captured your whole heart. It's hard to make sense of why they have to go.

On Christmas Day, while I was preparing a large holiday dinner, a dear friend ran into my house and told me my cat was lying in the driveway and wasn't moving.

My cat was my best friend. We went everywhere together. I lived in San Francisco, and from a very young age, I taught him to walk on a leash through the city streets. We went grocery shopping together. Rock climbing. We'd even go to weddings. Everywhere I went, he went too.

When I ran outside, I found him alive but unable to move his back legs. Having grown up on a ranch, I assumed he'd been hit by a car or been in a bad fight. I gently scooped him up, and a friend drove us to the nearest vet.

Upon arrival, we were told no veterinarians were on staff – everyone was on holiday. Only vet technicians were available. They took him in and discovered a large blood clot blocking circulation to his back legs. When I asked what could be done, they said surgery – but the nearest surgeon was three hours away. It was Christmas Day.

I was heartbroken. They put him on oxygen and tried to stabilize him with blood thinners. I paced around the block, talking to a friend, trying to think. When I came back, the techs told me his lungs were beginning to fill with blood. The most humane thing to do was let him go.

I couldn't believe what I was hearing. Letting him go felt impossible. They showed me the X-rays. There was a lot of blood.

With a heavy heart, I made one thing clear: If they were going to euthanize him, they were not taking him to a back room without me. They would bring him to me, with all their equipment, and we would do it together.

I placed him on my lap. Half of his body was still warm and alive. The other half was cold and still. Yet he had willpower – right up until his final moment, he fought to live. I talked to him and told him how much I loved him, and that this was what we had to do. As the tech brought the needle close to his leg, he tried to leap from my arms. I pulled him back, held him tight, and whispered: "I'm sorry, buddy. I love you."

Within seconds, his heart stopped. His body went limp. And then something profound happened. Everything I had ever been taught about death – every flatline on every TV screen – told me that when the heart stops, it's over. Time to grieve and move on.

But that's not what I experienced.

Even though his body was no longer moving, I felt his presence fill the entire room. I was surrounded, enveloped by his energy. In that moment, I knew there was more to death than what I'd been told. More to life than what I'd been shown. He was my awakening. My heart had to be broken by his death to be broken open.

After some time, the vet technicians returned with the official paperwork – cause of death. I looked down at the page and froze.

Feline Aortic Thromboembolism. F.A.T.E.

Guess what my cat's name was!

Kismet.

It means fate, or destiny – a word found in five different languages, pronounced the same way, meaning the same thing across all of them. It was fate that I met him. And it was his death that compelled me to pursue my purpose.

His passing ignited in me a deep desire to understand spirit – the nature of consciousness beyond this physical body. He propelled me to seek initiation into the Mystery Schools and explore the deeper mysteries of the universe. He opened a door, and I walked through it.

I now see him as one of my spirit guides, who sacrificed his physical body so I could learn that life extends beyond this form – and that each moment in this temporal, physical state is something to be cherished.

Thank you, Kismet.

Kismet taught me that death is not an ending – it is a threshold. And it was a teacher named Gareth Knight who gave language to what I had felt in that waiting room:

> The physical world is a definite stage in spiritual development – a gate one must pass through. By birth we come into this world, and by death we go out of it. Birth and death are two sides of the same coin: when one dies physically, one is born into the higher worlds, and when one is born physically, from the perspective of the higher worlds, one has died.
>
> – Gareth Knight

The goal of the esoteric student is to learn to use this gate consciously – to bring greater awareness of spirit into the flesh, to bring heaven to earth. This is what I now teach and share with others, and the state of being I live and embody.

There are many mysteries waiting to be unlocked when the soul is ready to open the door. We create contracts with one another to awaken and inspire each other. Sometimes those contracts appear painful – but the pain comes from not yet understanding. Used correctly, that pain can propel you into higher awareness.

And if you are reading this, perhaps it is no accident. Perhaps your own Kismet – whatever form it has taken – has already been nudging you toward the door. The only question is whether you are ready to walk through it.

Life is full of mystery. Often we aren't able to see the larger meaning in our experiences until later, when we look back and see how life flowed differently afterward. As Ashley shares, it is the goal of the awakened Soul to choose these transitional moments consciously so that we can use them to their full potential. The more aware we are of the opportunities presenting themselves to us, the more easily we can move forward without so much pain or suffering.

Many people experience that their love for their pet led them on a life path they never anticipated. Those experiences of awakening are often marked by pain or loss, which catapults them onto a mission driven by love. One of the great purposes of spiritual initiation in an ancient lineage is to help us access deeper levels of awakening without requiring these hard "wake-up calls." Initiation opens doors to greater potential, and then it is up to us to decide whether to walk through them.

One of the most profound and important lessons we can take from life is that there is always something more beneath the surface appearance, although the lessons might not be immediately clear to us. This is what esoterics, metaphysics and hermetics is all about. If we can rise above the current of our thoughts and emotions, we have the opportunity to connect with this greater message and entertain the possibility that there might be something for us in our difficult experiences besides just pain. There might be a gateway to our own healing, growth or awakening. And our pets might be ushering us through that doorway.

You Are More Than Your Experiences

You are not your thoughts and emotions. You experience thoughts. You experience emotions. They are not who you are. You are much more.

The Mystery School tradition teaches that we humans are made of three main bodies: Physical Body, Soul Body and Spirit Body. Within those three main parts exist the aspects of our physical, mental and emotional health and well-being. They are intricately related and interdependent. You may have heard this idea before. It wasn't a new concept to me when I started studying esoterics, metaphysics and hermetics with my spiritual mentors: Gudni Gudnason, founder of the Modern Mystery School, and Dave Lanyon and Hideto Nakagome, all Sovereign lineage holders in the Mystery School lineage of King Salomon. What was new was the invitation to take that contemplation deeper. When I learned a more nuanced understanding of the important way these three aspects of us are intertwined and how we can work with them, it brought a completely new perspective to why this is so important to understand in the realm of healing.

In the modern era, we have been conditioned to separate our spiritual well-being from our physical well-being. This was never the case in ancient times. It used to be taught that spiritual and physical were both important parts of our health, two sides of the same coin. Science was validly both physical (chemistry) and metaphysical (alchemy). Now, although exposure to and research in quantum physics is growing by leaps and bounds, physical science is still considered the only "real" science by many medical practitioners and others in the world as a whole.

That is changing, though! We are starting to awaken once again to who we are in all our multifaceted dimensions. It is an exciting time to be on the planet!

As a result of this separation made between our Physicality and Spirituality, our Soul (our emotions and mental state) has suffered. I see this as a contributing factor to the increasing stress and anxiety manifesting in society as a whole. This could be understood as a disorder of the Soul. The remedy is to reconnect with the core essence of who we are so that we can become whole again as we live our lives successfully in this physical world.

The first step is to calm the body and mind so you can experience some stillness. From that stillness can arise greater clarity about who you are, what you want, what is really important to you, and what will be helpful for you to achieve your dreams, goals and healing.

I invite you to explore the stories you hold about your life, about who you are, and about what you are truly capable of. All these stories become beliefs that then become the scaffolding of your reality. What story are you telling yourself right now about your current situation? Take a moment to write that down. Consider the following prompts:

What is the story I have about my pet's cancer?

What is the story I have about myself in the context of my pet's cancer?

Now ask yourself if there is a different way you could write that script that would better support you and your pet. That may be very difficult if you are feeling stressed right now. Stress narrows your focus and makes it harder for you to see the big picture. Take a few deep breaths, maybe go for a walk, do something to relax. Then come back and try to imagine the following.

Instead of asking, "Why is this happening TO me?" ask, "Why is this happening FOR me?"

Imagine there is a bigger picture. One that you aren't seeing right now. I'm not going to ask you to try and find the silver lining in this. It's unlikely you will be able to authentically do that right now. I *am* inviting you to see if you can connect with a higher purpose for your own life.

What are you passionate about? What brings you a feeling of fulfillment? What connects you with a feeling of peace, passion or purpose? Do you feel that you are here for a reason? If so, can you describe it? If you can think of something, write it down. Then, try to connect this journey with your pet into that bigger mission.

Don't worry if you can't. It's okay. You aren't broken. You are becoming. It is possible to reconnect with yourself, with that inner core. For now, just imagine there is something bigger than you – a story beyond the things you are thinking and feeling now, even if you can't see it yet. Entertain the idea. Let yourself imagine.

The mind drives us toward places using fear as the motivator. The heart calls us to be at peace and seek our JOY. The heart often knows the answer the mind can't grasp or refuses, often in frustration. Everything good in your life has started with the desires of your heart, not your mind. When you understand what you want based on your heart's desire, you move your Will. And it is through the Will that we can carefully command the mind in motion.

– Dave Lanyon, Sovereign Ipsissimus,
teacher of hermetics and lineage holder in the
Mystery School lineage of King Salomon

You came here with a purpose. You could call that a Soul Purpose. Have you ever thought about your Soul Purpose? This is the plan that was laid out before you were born, like your life blueprint. In this blueprint is recorded the plan for your life. Some of us are born with a conscious sense of that. I knew from a very young age that I was going to be a veterinarian, for example. I know that is one part of my Soul Purpose. Many people, though, don't have a conscious awareness of that yet.

When we live in alignment with our Soul Purpose we feel at ease, even during trials and trouble. If you had a lived understanding of those things and you were fulfilling that purpose through your daily life, you would feel peaceful. You would experience joy, a deep indwelling sense of uplifted well-being, as you were living your life in alignment with who you really are, not based on what others expect from you, how others define you, or what society says you should be doing. You might still do all the same things, but you would be doing them because they fulfilled you. You would experience this joy throughout the activities and events of your life.

There is a great amount of healing that arrives when we connect with the essence of who we are, underneath the demands of daily life, our career, and our other responsibilities. In our busy lives we often don't give ourselves time to contemplate these bigger questions: Who am I? What is my purpose? We don't often create time to nurture our Soul, which connects us to that level of understanding.

It is important, in your Whole-Being Wellness lifestyle, to do something every day to nurture your Soul.

Things that nurture your Soul:

- Meditation.
- Contemplating that you have a Soul Purpose.
    - What if this were true?
    - Would it help me?
    - Would it change how I am choosing to live my life?

- Helping other people also nurtures your Soul.
    - The trick is to help others from a full cup so that you are able to give without getting depleted. That requires taking care of yourself first.
    - The other trick is doing it without expecting anything in return.

People often talk about what they would do if they knew they only had a short time to live. In many cases, the answer people will give if they are more spiritually aware has more to do with their Soul Purpose. These are things that they feel are deeply important to them or which they feel passionate about. I'm talking about more than taking vacations or quitting your job so you don't have to work so hard. I'm referring to the things that fill you up, that energize you. Endeavors that make your life feel like it has meaning. These are often related to the legacy you wish to leave.

When you are living each day in fulfillment of these bigger picture things, you feel less stressed. You will still experience challenges, but you will be energized by the work you are doing. You will not seek to escape life. You will lean into the effort because it will bring you a sense of fulfillment.

Your Pet Is Your Partner

When you are in alignment, you are at peace on the inside. You feel less stress. Your pet benefits from this.

They might also be partners in this bigger mission. Maybe you have a service animal and you visit the sick and elderly. Maybe they help you stay grounded as you make these moves to fulfill your higher purpose. Maybe animals have something to do with your life purpose. Maybe the experiences you have with your pets create opportunities for you to open to your life purpose more deeply – they connect you with people who are part of this life path, or they help you open your heart so you can feel life more completely and connect with the deeper aspects of yourself.

What if your pet is teaching you something about life? This is a huge piece for many of the clients I see. The people who come to see me after their pet has been diagnosed with cancer are very bonded to their pet. You might even say they have a Soul connection or a bond that goes deeper than superficial appearances. It is common for people to feel a very deep connection to their pet or to feel that their pet was "sent to them." Our pets can teach us many things. They can invite us out of our shell. They are often excellent points of human connection, opening conversation and connection with others. They can teach us about the present moment. They can teach us about enjoying life. They can teach us about acceptance and loyalty.

One of the most powerful healings our pets can invite us into is to remind us that we are lovable. This can begin to heal deep wounds that we carry within ourselves related to lack of self-worth or self-love. They can remind us, through our love of them, that we are capable of opening our heart and loving. Their unconditional acceptance can be an invitation to give some attention to these parts of us that need healing.

When we understand our self-worth and that we are lovable, we are able to step into our Soul Purpose in important ways that are not accessible to us otherwise. You may choose to explore this in any way that is available to you. There are many self-help books about this topic since it is such a common limitation we place on ourselves. In my experience, self-help books and mental/emotional work have their limits in this area. Why? Because while much of the thought process can be addressed, this is a deeper Soul-level issue because it has to do with forgetting who you really are.

If you remembered who you REALLY are, you would love yourself. Not in an egotistical way in which you are better than other people, but in a way that reflects an experience of your wholeness and an understanding that we are all worthy of Love. If you are interested in metaphysical healing that gets to the level of your Soul, the best first step I have experienced to help you begin to heal these deeper levels and awaken the realization of your Soul Purpose is, once again, a Life Activation. This is the first step, and it opens the door to greater potential and next steps. For those who are open to exploring this deeper healing work, I find nothing more rewarding than supporting them in that journey.

Part III Takeaway
Soul Health

Focus on Soul Body Health

- Do one thing every day for mental and emotional balance.
- Focus on what you can control.
- Exercise your power to choose the stories you entertain.
- Tend to your own mental/emotional imbalances as well as your pet's.
- Try out new ways to support yourself and your pet energetically.

Activity Ideas

- If you need to, make an appointment with a therapist to help you process what is going on with your pet and also within yourself.
- Make a list of three things you are grateful for every day. Keep a running list and visit this whenever you are having a hard day. Read these out loud to your pet, as you are connecting with gratitude.
- Spend five minutes in one sensory absorption session with your pet, letting your mind rest in the present moment.
    - Go outside and connect with nature – see, smell, hear and touch.
    - Listen to your favorite relaxing song with your eyes closed. Really listen. Classical music is excellent for this, and your pet will enjoy it.
- Laugh! Laughter is the best medicine for the Soul.
    - Read a feel-good book or watch a funny movie.

- Laugh with friends, family and your pet.
- Make a playdate for your dog and enjoy the fun!

- Meditate with your pet.
- Snuggle with your pet and allow yourself to simply enjoy their presence.
- Schedule a healing session for you and your pet with a trained metaphysical/energy healing practitioner you trust.

Esoteric Contemplation Invitation

- Contemplate what is really important to you in life. Allow yourself to move beyond physical things like money and health.
  - How do you want to feel in your life? What do you want?
  - Often, we want what we want because we believe it will make us feel a certain way. For example, when I have __________, then I will finally be/feel __________.
  - Is there another way you could connect with that emotion or state of being right now?
- Reflect on what brings you a sense of meaning and purpose.
- If someone asked you what your life purpose is, what would you say?
- What is the legacy you want to create?

PART 4

THE SPIRIT

A large body of evidence indicates that spirituality is associated with better health outcomes, including greater longevity, coping, and quality of life.[77]

– Journal of the American Medical Association, 2022

Spirituality as a Path to Wholeness

While I have a deep interest and passion for veterinary integrative oncology and two decades of clinical experience in the topics already discussed in this book, my most driving passion is for the topic of spiritual health and healing. That is the focus of this last section.

I am uniquely qualified to speak to this topic because of my training and life experience. There are many board-certified veterinary oncologists who can help you navigate the terrain of conventional cancer therapy. There are many veterinarians well-trained in holistic, alternative medicine and integrative medicine modalities who can assist you in appropriate fresh food feeding options, acupuncture, herbal medicine and even energy medicine interventions. But few also have the depth of training and experience I do with universal spirituality, and who practice this on a regular basis as a way of life.

There are powerful, untapped resources to support your well-being and your ability to transform the trouble you are experiencing now into something more than just survival.

I can open new avenues for you to consider, while also being uniquely experienced as a medical veterinary oncologist still working in a clinical setting, helping real patients and pet parents navigate their cancer journey. This is the main reason I wrote this book – to open doors of awareness and well-being.

Before I dive into my experience, perspectives and approach, some clarifications are necessary. As you are likely in a delicate emotional place, which can increase sensitivity and reactivity, I also want to address common resistances right up front so that you can relax. Please know I have immense compassion for you and the fact that all of us have different beliefs. That is part of the human condition on this planet. It also makes life interesting and is the fertile ground upon which we can respectfully explore new concepts, bringing us into new levels of understanding about ourselves and the human condition.

Often, when the words Spirituality or God come up, the mind immediately goes to religion. That is not what I am talking about; religion is a different topic altogether. The world has many religions, and I am not aiming to tell you what to believe, make anyone wrong, or disturb the foundation of nurturing practices that support you. I simply want to begin a conversation about what unites us as a human race.

Spirituality is something that we all have in common. We are all spiritual beings having a physical experience. We have also all been brought up in different cultures and societies that have formed the foundation of our personal beliefs and behaviors.

Religions tend to divide us, as they focus on separating people into groups and tribes based on differences in beliefs. Often those differences can be minor and still result in divisiveness, even between sects of the same religion. Additionally, everyone has a different personal relationship with religion and the word "God."

I know many people who are deeply religious and find great comfort in their religious teachings, dogmas, ceremonies, rites and practices. I have no interest in dismantling beliefs that serve you and help you live a better, more compassionate and joyful life. I want that to be clear from the start.

On the other hand, I also know many people who have had traumatic experiences related to religion. Those experiences have altered them so deeply that they have turned away from religion – and, in many cases, everything that it stands for, including their relationship with a greater creative power, the idea of "God," and their own spirituality.

Then there are those who are agnostic and those who are atheist. Some like to label people as either "religious" or "non-religious."

I am not interested in further dividing us, or encouraging judgmentalism. The world has enough of that. It isn't helpful, and you are already in a fragile state. I do, however, wish to present some ways of thinking about who you are and what this life is that might expand the current story you have about life. My intention is to open up the opportunity for you to connect more fully with yourself and your relationship with the

Universal Source of Creation, which you might call God. You might have a different name. Or you might choose not to name it at all, preferring to think of it as an energy.

Spirituality, as I am using the term here, has to do with your relationship with the part of you and the universe that is more than your physical body, your mind, and your thoughts and emotions. It is the part of your experience that both includes and transcends your past, present and future circumstances in this human life. That spiritual relationship influences everything in your life, everything you do, and everything you experience, whether you believe that now or not. This is a fundamental part of being human. Healthy spirituality is foundational to human thriving and to experiencing joy through this journey of life.

The more you can open and connect to something larger than the limited sphere of your body, mind and emotions, the more peace, power and potential you will have to turn challenges into opportunities for growth and healing. You will be more able to see the beauty in life, even when things feel hard. And you will be more able to enjoy the precious moments that you have with those you love, including your pet.

This last section of the book will crack the door open to that conversation, letting a little Light into this journey when you are inundated with physical science, medicine, opinions and hard decisions. Its goal is to bring hope amidst the overwhelm, worry, fear, grief, anger and all the other heavy emotions. I'm also excited to connect with those of you who are already living in awareness of your spiritual nature but who may be looking for something deeper – a way to grow into a greater understanding, transcending obstacles that hold you back from where you want to be in your life.

What if one of your pet's gifts to you was to lead you on a journey that ultimately connected you more closely with your life purpose, greater fulfillment, transformation and joy? That might seem impossible to imagine right now. It might even feel offensive, if you are really in the midst of deep despair. I understand that. No one wants to suffer, and I don't believe it is necessary for growth. Often, though, we do suffer. So when we suffer, we might as well grow. I assure you it has happened for people I know. It happened for me. There is even a term for it in psychology: "post-traumatic growth." I'm not trained to speak on the deeper psychology of that. I am merely here to help you entertain that potential by opening up the conversation of spirituality as a resource to support you through this cancer caregiver journey.

Why? Because we write our own story. We are the ones who choose what to do with the experiences in front of us. While it might be a long time before you are able to come out the other side and see the Light at the end of the tunnel, it also might be that you are ready. You must honor your journey and take the time you need to heal. But please know there is hope. This too shall pass, and you are stronger than you know.

All true healing is ultimately
the restoration of wholeness
between the individual and the Divine.

– Dion Fortune, psychologist

Chapter 13

What if There Is Something More?

Just as research on Mental/Emotional practices that originated in spiritual traditions has increased in the past two decades, so has research studying the importance of spiritual health in cancer patient caregivers. In ancient traditions, spirituality was always an essential component of healing. Traditional healers always recognized that Spirit is an inseparable part of our human health and wellness.

It is exciting to see the movement back toward integrating spirituality into wellness care in conventional medicine circles. Many approaches are being investigated to better define the factors that positively influence what is termed "post-traumatic growth" in pediatric cancer survivorship, especially related to parents of children diagnosed with cancer. One of the aims of this is to improve psychosocial oncology care.

Despite many research studies identifying the importance of spiritual care in oncology care discussions, studies show that very few oncologists incorporate this in their care discussions.[78, 79, 80] This may be due to a lack of clarity about how to best implement these discussions, a lack of training, a lack of time, and challenges navigating intense emotions.[81, 82] This highlights a huge area of opportunity in improving our oncology patient care, not only in human medicine but in our veterinary oncology arena as well.

Research in spirituality is fraught with challenges due to the complexities of the ways individuals connect with, or do not connect with, spirituality. In addition, in order to conduct a clinical trial, measurable, quantifiable variables must be evaluated and compared. But how do you measure the quality of someone's internal subjective experience? The only way to do that is to measure the outward manifestations of that private inner experience.

While I do not aim to focus heavily on the psychology of spirituality, it is important to present some research to provide some grounding for the journey I am inviting you on in the remainder of this book. For those of us who are logical and strongly attached to "proof," this is one way to open the door to understanding the complexities of the human experience. That can build an appreciation for how much we still have to learn about effectively creating greater inner stability, peace of mind, balance and connection amidst the ever-changing circumstances and inevitable pains life presents to us.

In terms of psychology, spirituality and religion are often grouped together. However, many people would say they are spiritual but not religious, and many others would say they are religious but not spiritual. So spirituality, in research settings, has been evaluated separately from religion. For this purpose, spirituality has been defined as "the search for meaning, purpose, and connection with self, others, the universe, and ultimate reality, however one understands it, which may or may not be expressed through religious forms or institutions."[83]

Studies suggest that higher spiritual well-being in cancer caregivers correlates with improved quality of life, lower perceived burden, and increased likelihood of post-traumatic growth.[84, 85, 86] In other words, higher spirituality correlates with an increased likelihood of experiencing positive growth through coping with and overcoming the challenges of the cancer caregiver journey. Conversely, studies show negative manifestations of spirituality are associated with decreased health outcomes. For example, a negative sense of God is associated with increased anxiety and depression in oncology patients.[87] This highlights the variability in spiritual health among individuals and its impact on well-being.

I am not a trained clinical therapist or psychologist and do not work in this arena. However, given my role as a veterinary oncologist, I encounter the traumatic material of my clients on a daily basis. I see firsthand how different people navigate the cancer journey – and some have far more difficulty than others. So how do we practically apply this? Are there specific interventions that can support you as you navigate the cancer journey with your pet that you can do today, on your own? The answer is yes.

A 2019 study found a simple practice resulted in significant improvement in the well-being of mothers whose children had been diagnosed with cancer.[88] This is something practical that you could start exploring on your own right now to see if it helps you. This practice will be especially helpful to you if you already have a positive relationship with God, or some other creative force that you believe exists. If you don't, then you could write a letter to the universe, or whatever feels authentic for you. In this study, mothers of children diagnosed with cancer were asked to spend 20 minutes each day writing a letter to God expressing their sincere desires or wishes, without any worry or stress – just free-form writing. This practice resulted in decreased anxiety compared to a group that simply journaled their daily schedule and tasks for 20 minutes.

When one starves the soul and spirit,
they will never find inner peace or true lasting satisfaction.
When life is only the physical and the mind,
the soul and spirit suffer, and you suffer for it.

– Dave Lanyon, Sovereign Ipsissimus,
teacher of hermetics and lineage holder
in the Mystery School lineage of King Salomon
You Are Not Perfect the Way You Are

Reconnecting with Your Essence

People may reject spirituality or doubt the idea that there is a spiritual aspect, foundation or dimension to not only life but to each one of us, for many different reasons. Maybe you are one of those people. Maybe you aren't but you know some who are.

Some people grew up without a spiritual aspect to their upbringing, or in a family that rejected it, and they adopted those beliefs. Some say they have never experienced any evidence that there is anything more than the physical. More people, in my experience, once had a relationship with God and then chose to reject that part of life due to their life experiences.

In my 20 years of teaching in yoga, esoterics, philosophy, and now in the work I do as a spiritual mentor in the Mystery School lineage, I have met many people who have had some kind of negative experience related to religion that has caused them to reject that part of their life and everything related to it. I understand.

I have met many who became angry with God after a life event that they could not process or refused to accept. Their anger at the circumstance resulted in an anger at God, who in their perspective failed to protect them or a loved one, failed to prevent suffering or death, or failed to answer a prayer. I also understand that.

I know many who have disconnected from the spiritual aspect of their existence because they rejected their experience of religion or the tenets of religious dogma that no longer felt aligned with their morals and a compassionate way of living in the world. I especially understand that.

I also know many who are highly spiritual and have no affiliation with any organized religion. They live a very rich spiritual life and feel a strong sense of connection to others, nature, a universal creative power, and their own inner divinity.

I also know people who, as I wrote previously, have a very strong religious affiliation and have found great peace, fulfillment and purpose in that organized system of faith. They find a deep comfort in their religious practices, and it has helped them weather many of life's trials and tribulations with grace.

These final chapters are not about religion. They are about You.

No matter where you fall on this spectrum, I'm going to invite you to entertain the question "What if there is something more?" Something more than you have been told, something more than you now believe, something more than your current experiences have provided to you. Something bigger than you have been willing to believe.

I'm not asking you to believe anything specific. I'm just asking you to entertain the possibility that you don't have all the answers, and that there might be even deeper levels of well-being, peace, stillness and joy available to you than you have yet experienced.

Why? Because no matter who you are, you limit yourself on some level. You limit your happiness, joy and peace through the way you think about yourself and your life and the universe – by the way you do or don't think about God.

Overcoming Limiting Beliefs

Think of the ways you limit yourself now. Let me take you back to the beginning of the book to the ways you could define yourself on this journey. Do you remember which one you resonated most strongly with?

- **Heart-Seeker:** You are searching for deeper meaning and connection, often finding it through your pet. *Yearning is awakening. You sense there's "something more" but are unsure how to access it. You find deep meaning through your pet. You are learning to use that love to open a door to greater purpose.*
- **Devoted Giver:** You struggle with self-worth but pour love and care into your pet. *You often neglect yourself but rise fiercely in devotion for those you love. Your love burns brightly for others – now you are learning to turn that love inward.*
- **Shaken Soul:** You had a foundation but feel lost after the cancer diagnosis. *You have some spiritual grounding but that has been destabilized by the cancer diagnosis. Your compass has been shaken, and you are seeking grounding and guidance. Once rooted, you are awakening to deeper layers of strength.*
- **Purpose-Driven Pathfinder:** You are a high-achieving, mission-oriented individual craving deeper alignment and clarity. *You are motivated and capable, but seeking a soul-aligned map for what's next. You have done the work and seek*

true alignment with a higher purpose. Mission-driven and ready, you are seeking to walk in full Soul alignment.

Now find the one you chose and ask yourself the questions associated with it.

Heart-Seeker:

- Do you believe your life has meaning without your pet?
- Are you someone who says, "I can't imagine living after my pet is gone"?

Your life matters. There is a way to connect with deeper meaning and life purpose. You yearn for that because deep down, your Soul knows this is true even if your mind doesn't accept it yet.

You came here with a purpose to fulfill. We all did. You are not an exception. You can remember. There is a way to remember, a path to help you reconnect with the meaning of life and with your life purpose. Do you believe that?

Devoted Giver:

- Do you believe you are worthy of love? Do you love yourself?
- In what ways do you limit yourself from receiving love from others?

You matter. You are important. Believing that doesn't make others less important. Loving yourself is possible. And it is extremely important. You just have to remember who you are, underneath all the stories you carry about yourself.

You have a bigger purpose, and loving yourself allows you to really love others the way you want to, deep down. There is an endless supply of love available to you. You yearn to fully embody that love, because it is a part of who you are. Love is not an emotion. Love is a force that runs through all of us. It runs through you.

When you reject love, when you don't accept it, you limit yourself. You are a beautiful being. Nobody is perfect, so you can let go of that ideation right now. Your true essence, your Spiritual Self, the one that existed before you were born into this life, is beauty and love and goodness. You could call that your Higher Self.

As you accept that, you expand your capacity to care for others. And that allows you to step more fully into your Higher Self and the life you came here to live. When you are whole, you have a full cup. You can give without getting depleted.

Shaken Soul:

- Do you believe you are being punished in some way by a higher power?
- Do you feel betrayed or abandoned by God?
- Has your faith in life and the universe been rattled because of the pain of this experience?
- Do you feel uncertain about how to move forward?

You are not alone, even if it feels that way now. There is a higher order at play, and sometimes from our vantage point we can't see the bigger picture. That isn't to say this was "supposed to happen" – but it is happening. Maybe there is an opportunity within this pain, an opportunity to reconnect with your power. Perhaps it contains an invitation to no longer entertain the mindset of being a victim of the circumstances of your life. Instead, you can decide to embrace this opportunity to grow and ground yourself in the bigger picture. You can use this opportunity to connect more deeply with yourself and explore your potential even more earnestly.

While there is something bigger than your small self, you are ultimately the driver of your life. You are here to make choices, to create something out of the chaos in front of you. And sometimes that feels chaotic or ungrounding. That is okay. There is a way to live connected spiritually, and fully empowered to participate in the life you are co-creating with God/Universe/Source.

Life presents us with endless cycles of pain and pleasure. There is a way to ground yourself in knowing there is a bigger picture, even if you can't see it now – and to journey into the future with more stability and peace so that you stay balanced through the ups and downs of life.

That is a process. It doesn't happen overnight. Sometimes, looking back, you might see that out of your biggest challenges have come your greatest growths. You never grow if you don't have the opportunity to push yourself beyond your current limits. Your love for your pet can drive you to push yourself to be more than you are today. You are stronger than you think you are, and you are never alone.

Purpose-Driven Pathfinder:

- Are you frustrated at the lack of control you feel around your pet's cancer diagnosis?
- Do you find yourself refusing to accept the situation in front of you?
- Are you driven to seek out every possibility to the point that you begin feeling overwhelmed and confused?
- Are you looking for a map to success?

You are self-motivated and not afraid of hard work. You often take the weight of the world on your shoulders and can carry the burden with grace. But deep down, you feel you are missing something. You have an inner yearning that knows there is another piece of the puzzle that hasn't been revealed to you yet, so you are always looking for more. You have likely taken "all the workshops" and read "all the books." You've been to therapy, tried biohacking, and taken every training you could find.

Now, you don't have all the answers. That doesn't sit well. The "more" for you is going to be hard to hear. It is surrender. Not in the sense of giving up, but in the sense of letting go – connecting with the flow of nature and the flow of the universe. You need to balance your drive to "do" with the necessity to "just be" in the moment. There is a huge quantum field of potential that exists within each moment. When you open up to that flow, what you have been searching for has an opportunity to come to you in a new way – not through your mind but through your heart, your Spirit.

The key you have been yearning for has to do with learning how to connect with the field of potential you could call God or Universe, and then bringing that through you into your life. That is the realm of miracles. While others reading this book might laugh and call that silly, or even wrong, you feel it is true. Your Soul knows it, even if your mind doesn't accept it now.

This is the realm of the Alchemists, the original scientists, who transformed and created in a different way. And there is a path that has been preserved for millennia for those who want to step into that way of living. They learn to work in cooperation with the Divine to make the world a better place and invite miracles into this life, defying the laws of nature and medicine. This is the realm of Spirit, and it is so much more than thinking positive and holding intentions. There is a science to it.

When you live this way with integrity, you always remember that there is a higher order. You understand you do not have the right to interfere with the free will of others. You always work to help and to heal. You also remember that there is a natural flow to life and death. In the context of your journey with your pet after a cancer diagnosis, you learn all you can – and then use all the tools at your disposal to give them every opportunity to heal.

You do this not because you fear death, but because you honor life. You know that in the end, death is also part of this experience, and that your pet does not cease to exist after their physical body expires.

In this higher state of awareness, you know it isn't for you to dictate how your pet responds to treatment. So you surrender to the Divine as you continue to work to help and heal. You accept that what you want may not always be what plays out in the dance of life. But knowing you did your best, you are at peace. And you move on to the next task, knowing your Soul and Spirit are aligned with what is Good and that you are living your mission, driven by Love. Love flows through you. It isn't "you" that makes miracles. It is Love.

Love knows when to help and when to let nature take its course.

Do you connect with anything I said above? What resistances are coming up for you? These places we hold resistance are where we have room to grow. It is best to just play at the edges of those resistances. Question what you don't believe yet. Measure that against what you do believe. Ask yourself if what you do believe is serving you. Give yourself permission to question your own beliefs, to test them. Maybe they served you in the past but now they are limiting you. In the end, Love is the main point I want to drive home here.

- Notice where you are not connecting to love for yourself, and therefore seek it elsewhere.

- Notice where you are not connecting with love in your relationships with other humans.
- Notice where you are not connecting with love from God, or the Universal Creative force that runs through all created things, so you seek it elsewhere.

Love for your pet is Good. But your pet isn't meant to replace the Love you experience from these three – only to enhance your life, to bring it greater depth, to give you another avenue to express Love and care for another being. The love we experience from our pets is special; for some, it may be the only experience of unconditional love they have had. That makes the thought of losing them exceptionally painful. It might even feel unbearable.

But what if you could use that love to awaken the love that lives inside of you? What if you could use that love to nurture that potential in healthy relationships with other humans? Wouldn't that be the most powerful gift your pet could leave you? It would, because Love connects us to the universal flow of the Divine, God, Spirit. And that is most definitely real.

CHAPTER 13 CHECK-IN

Daily Activity

- Each day, for 20 minutes, write a letter to God, the Universe or Source expressing your sincere desires or wishes for you and your pet, without any worry or stress.
- Relax and let this be a free-form flow of consciousness writing.

Journal Exercise

Journal the answers to the questions associated with the caregiver type you connect with most strongly.

Heart-Seeker: You are searching for deeper meaning and connection, often finding it through your pet.

- What is most important to you right now?
- What do you want to accomplish in your life? What are your dreams?

Devoted Giver: You struggle with self-worth but pour love and care into your pet.

- List 10 good qualities about yourself.
- Keep this list with you in a place you can see it.
- What activities do you enjoy? Why?
- How can you bring more of these into your life?

Shaken Soul: You had a foundation but feel lost after the cancer diagnosis.

- List 10 of your strengths.
- Keep this list with you in a place you can see it.
- List three ways you feel connected with something bigger than yourself – God, Universe or Source – or ways you could try to feel that.
- For example, it might be in the awe you feel when you are in the mountains, out in nature, by the ocean or stargazing. It might be in the laughter and innocence of children. It might be in prayer or meditation.

Purpose-Driven Pathfinder: You are a high-achieving, mission-oriented individual craving deeper alignment and clarity.

- What is working well for you in your life right now?
- What do you want to learn more about?
- What areas of your life bring you the most meaning, interest and sense of fulfillment? Why?

The imagination of a man is a great factor in medicine; for it may produce diseases in man and in animals, and it may cure them.

– Paracelsus, Swiss physician, alchemist and philosopher
De Imaginatione

Chapter 14

Intuition, Connection and the Power of Prayer

We are powerful, and often unaware of the true scope of those powers that can help us move through life with more ease and grace. Some people may seem particularly psychic or gifted, but the truth is that we all have intuition, and this is a power we can develop. We can learn how to use these powers and energy to connect to ourselves, our pets, other humans and the Divine. One of the most important and ancient spiritual technologies is prayer, which has been proven to work. Let us take a look at these powers and how you can develop them.

Intuition

What is intuition? Intuition is also sometimes called "psychic senses" or your "sixth sense." Pets are very psychic. I am sure there have been times you feel your pet just "knows" something. They can sense or even see things that you don't.

I know many of you reading this book feel your pet communicates with you at another level. They seem to know what you are thinking or feeling. There are physical ways we have already talked about to explain this, and there is research to show that animals can smell our emotions through chemokines (chemicals) that our body emits when we are experiencing certain emotions. Animals also have intuitive senses.

Growing up, I had a cat named Topaz, who would often stare into the corners of the room and track with her eyes things I couldn't see. She would chirp as she did this, like she would chirp when she was watching the birds out the window. Maybe you have even seen things out of the corner of your eye, and then when you move your head to look, there is nothing there. We often make stories to write off these perceptions. But there are energies we can perceive with our intuitive senses. We can learn to develop them.

You already have intuition operating in your life. Everyone does. You get a "gut feeling." You just "know" something you can't explain. There is a great benefit in learning how you receive these intuitive hits, which are really messages from Spirit – from your Higher Self, from God and from the angelic realm. When you begin to trust these intuitions, life takes on a whole new dimension, because you are able to receive guidance in more ways.

Your intuitive senses are linked with your physical senses: sight, smell, taste, touch and hearing. When you develop your intuitive senses, you are able to communicate with them more clearly. The human-animal bond strengthens and takes on a new dimension. You can practice opening up your spiritual senses with your pet in many ways. You want to do this slowly and in a balanced and safe way, and the techniques can be fun games.

One of my favorite ways to do this, opening up your inner hearing, is to sit and really practice listening deeply. This technique is often taught in mindfulness training, but I was also taught it as a practice in my Mystery School training to open up spiritual senses. It is a practice of deep listening. You can do this exercise with your pet and they will likely find it very relaxing. Sit quietly with your pet and close your eyes. Listen closely to the beat of your heart. Then expand your attention out to sounds you can hear in the room, then in the rest of the house, then outside the house. See how far out you can hear sounds. Maybe you can hear birds or the sound of traffic far off in the distance. Then bring your attention to the sounds you hear back in, until you are again listening only to the sound of your own heart beating, letting all other sounds fall away. I particularly enjoy doing this practice outside in nature.

Here is a fun game you can practice to open up your ability to perceive information by touch. Take a crystal or semi-precious gemstone in your hand such as quartz, rose quartz, amethyst, lapis, carnelian, citrine, aventurine or malachite. Close your eyes and see how much information you can pick up. Can you sense the color? Do you feel any sensations in areas of your physical body? Do any emotions or thoughts come up? As you practice, you will become more familiar with how you pick up and receive information. A lot of this practice is learning to trust what you are receiving – to trust yourself.

A Note of Care

On Trust:

Many of us have had experiences that make it hard for us to trust others, ourselves or a higher power. I understand and recognize this is a common struggle. To move beyond it requires healing. If you have a hard time with trust, this next section may be more challenging for you. I assure you, difficulty with trust can be healed, though it may require working with healers to support you, and a healthy dose of your own will to do it. In order to heal, you have to want to heal. But if you do want to heal, anything is possible.

Notice I didn't say healing will definitely happen. I said possibility exists. Your choices and actions open those possibilities. Because you are connected to an infinite field of possibility. Some in the modern era call that the quantum field; some call that God.

On Words:

Going forward, I am going to use the word "God" for ease of communication and flow of reading. If that word triggers you or makes it hard for you to read what I am presenting for your consideration, please just substitute a different word on your own. Some suggestions are Universe, Source Field, Creative Energy and Spirit. "God" can be a tricky word because it has been used for so many human agendas, and so many wrongs have been committed in the name of that word that it can be a challenge for some. From my personal perspective, the word you use doesn't really matter. In the end, God is not something you can describe with any word. You can only experience God. Words merely point to ideas, to concepts.

You may have your own concepts attached to the word "God" that have been formed based on what you have been told by your family, religion, society and what you have decided for yourself based on your life experiences. We need to use words to communicate ideas. But, also, words are inadequate to describe phenomena that are beyond our human mind.

If the word "God" brings you comfort now, please use it. If it brings you pain, then please use a different word that authentically connects you to the idea that there is something bigger than you, something more expansive, a creative force that exists outside of the realm of your current understanding – maybe even your current beliefs.

There is a very important point I am trying to make here, and I would like for you to be able to receive it, even if you choose not to agree. I am not asking for agreement; I am merely inviting you to think differently, to entertain the possibility that there may be a different perspective. One that is also true.

Connection

You are connected to God. God is not separate from you. God flows through you when you choose Good and Love and to live in alignment with Universal Principles. When you genuinely care for others and work to help them, God moves through you.

Is that idea hard for you? For some it is. That's okay. You don't have to believe it. I invite you to simply ask the questions: "What if that were true? What if I believed that? Would it help me? Would it help me to think differently? Would it open up the potential for new experiences that would benefit my life and the lives of those around me?"

Maybe that statement isn't difficult for you at all. Maybe you are like many others and it inspires you. Something inside of you is sparked to life. It gives you permission to lean into that awareness in a way you have been yearning for. Maybe that statement rings true to everything you have already known and currently believe.

For me, this connection was always my experience. And I have memories long into my very early years. As a child I always felt a deep interconnection with God. "God." That was the word I was given. But to me, "God" was never a "person." My experience was that God was in everything I could see, sense, touch, feel and hear. God was also definitely not something or someone separate from me.

I was an individual, yes, but God, which felt like an expansive presence rather than a "person," was never separate from me. It was a force running through me and all created things. I could always go inside myself and touch that Source of comfort, peace and love. And God helped me. When I was in trouble, I would simply ask and help would come. I have many stories I could tell you.

This made me a very interesting student to have in elementary parochial school religion class because, even at that young age, I questioned the teacher when she would say things about God that didn't fit with my lived experience. I was told to keep quiet and not ask those kinds of questions. So I did. I was a good student.

Then I got older and "life happened." One day, something occurred that severed that connection. I was well and grown at the time, and the experience was very traumatic. It caused intense inner suffering – suffering that was especially difficult because no one else could see it or really understand it. For the first time in my life, I felt truly and completely alone in the world. I remember talking to someone at the time, and they said, "Everyone feels that way." I remember that made me really angry, because that was not how I had ever felt – and I knew that wasn't how it was supposed to be.

Eventually, I was able to connect with people who helped me heal that disconnection. It wasn't through medicine or psychology (I did that) or trauma therapy (I did that too) or yoga or breathing practices (I did that as well) or "rewiring my nervous system" through anything physical science accepts as real or true. It also definitely wasn't through "plant medicine" or psychedelics.

It was metaphysical. What does that mean? It means it was beyond the physical. What is beyond the physical? Energy, the quantum field of potential, and our Spirit and that Beautiful and Good phenomenon humans often call "God." Those who dislike the word "God" – often because of what humans have done in the name of that word – call it Universe, Source Field, or any other number of things.

While that experience was extremely painful and difficult, it allowed me to understand how many people actually *do* feel. Disconnected. I had the experience of feeling "alone," even when there were people around me. I felt depressed and anxious. I felt like my life had lost its meaning and its color.

Because of that journey, I also experienced that there is a way to reconnect. And now, I understand how to help other people in a way that I would never have understood, had I not had the experience myself.

Prior to that experience, I could not understand how someone could not believe in some kind of God. I couldn't really understand how someone could believe we were inherently separate from God either. I understood why someone might not believe the story about God that they have been told; I understood why some people have a hard time with religion. I understood why some people are afraid to not believe what they have been told they must believe in order to go to heaven when they die. But I really could not understand how anyone could believe there was not something bigger than this small "me" in this body we are living in. It hadn't been imaginable to me, a life like that.

Many traditions understand and teach that we are not separate from God, and we use many stories to try to wrap our conceptual human minds around something that is both real and also cannot be thought about or accurately described with words. It must be experienced to be known to us. It must be experienced to move beyond intellectual knowledge and a human story into a lived experience that brings personal understanding. To me, that is one of the most beautiful things about spiritual practice, and the traditions that facilitate our lived experience of that connection.

That there is a way for us to experience that connection is the greatest gift, even if we have yet to experience it. It is the greatest comfort to know we are never really alone, even when we might feel like we are. There is, truly, a whole army of assistance we have that we often can't perceive with our physical senses. We all have spiritual guides. There are angelic beings, and there is God – even though the ultimate nature of these phenomena may defy our human understanding.

We are able to work with these energies. You can call them beings. They do help us. And they, unlike us, have a bird's-eye view of the bigger picture of our life and spiritual blueprint. We can call on these forces to help us in our time of need. You can ask for help when you need comfort or clarity on how to make a decision. You can call in this assistance for healing support, and to be connected to the people who will be able to help you and your pet.

Prayer

A Personal Story About the Power of Prayer

A number of years ago, my best childhood friend's father was in a very severe motorcycle accident. He almost died. Through the miracle of modern medicine and the skill of doctors, he didn't die. He underwent extensive surgery to repair a severed aorta and many, many, many broken bones. Her father had an army of friends and family praying for his healing and his comfort. He healed. Completely. The most remarkable part of this story, and the reason I am sharing it, is that he experienced a lack of pain that was completely unbelievable and unexplainable. With the amount of injury his body was dealing with, he should have been in excruciating pain 24/7. He wasn't. And he wasn't a super-human type who had an unusually high pain threshold his entire life. That, to me, is one type of miracle. It is just one example of how prayer can have a tangible effect. The power of prayer is real.

The human mind is powerful. *We* are powerful. There are so many things I could share with you about that, but it isn't really the point of this book. The relevant thing I want to invite you to think more deeply about is how prayer does, and doesn't, work. I am going to offer you a way to think about prayer that may be totally different than how you have thought about it before.

Not from the perspective of science, but from the perspective of Spirit.

Sometimes we limit ourselves because we insist on black and white, when in truth there might be a both/and situation going on. Paradox makes us uncomfortable. That fact has led to a great many arguments and divisive behaviors, feeding a need to make other people wrong. I do not wish to make you wrong. What I do wish is to offer an opportunity for you to expand and refine beliefs and behaviors that may not be serving you in the best way anymore. As we are exposed to new information, we have the opportunity to grow, adjust and gain a wider perspective than the one we have held until now.

I said at the start of this book, "Information doesn't change people's belief systems. Experience does." What I have learned through my hermetic Mystery School training supports that: True understanding is the product of a process. It is not acquired through information alone. To move toward understanding, we take what we have learned, our knowledge, and USE it in our life. This application of our knowledge to our lived experience of life brings us understanding.

What I present here is information. That information will not become understanding for you until you try it out, if you choose to. Until you have an EXPERIENCE.

Information doesn't change belief systems. Experience does.

That is because experience is required for understanding, and then for understanding to inform new beliefs.

I am going to share with you one way to deepen your relationship with prayer. This may go against what you have been told or how you have been engaging with prayer up until now. Or you might feel relieved because it makes sense to your Soul and feels absolutely right.

God, as understood through hermetics, is not the abdication of responsibility by assigning work through prayer and requests to a separate being but is in fact the embracing of that responsibility as something to personally act on if one wants it improved. As I tell my students, pray only for that which you are willing to act on and God will work with and through you.

– Dave Lanyon, Sovereign Ipsissimus,
teacher of hermetics and lineage holder
in the Mystery School lineage of King Salomon
You Are Not Perfect the Way You Are

What if you only prayed for that which you were willing to work toward? "Let go and let God" is a popular phrase. It doesn't mean you don't do anything. It means you do everything you can do and you let go of attachment to the outcome. For me, that does not negate faith. *Trust*, however, may actually be a better word. You pray. You do everything that is within your power. And you let go. You Trust. Let me expand on that idea for a moment.

For example, it would not make sense to pray for perfect healing of a broken bone and then not go to the doctor to have the bone set properly. Praying isn't asking God or some higher power to do something so that you are relieved of responsibility to take the actions that are available to you. God acts through the people and circumstances available to us in this world we live in. And God acts through you.

It is like the story you have probably heard before of a man trapped in a flood who prays to God for help. The water rises up through the floors of his house and he climbs up and up to escape the water until he is standing on the roof, praying to God to save him from drowning. A boat comes by and the person on the boat says, "Grab my hand, climb in, and we can row to safety." The man says, "No! God will save me!" The floodwaters rise and he climbs higher. A helicopter flies by and they throw down a rope and say, "Grab the rope and hang on tight. We will pull you up and fly to safety." And the man says, "No! God will save me!"

You know the story. The floodwaters rise and the man drowns. When he meets God in heaven he asks God, "Why didn't you save me?" God replies, "I tried. I sent you a boat and a helicopter and you refused the help I sent."

As a practical example, you don't pray for a new job and then sit on your couch watching TV and not go out and interview. That is disrespecting God and disrespecting yourself.

I am aware that, in some circles, acting in support of a prayer you have sent to God is seen as heretical. I have never understood that. As both a logical and spiritual person, that makes no sense to me. We did not come here to be inert, swept away by the current of whatever comes toward us. We came here to live life, learn and experience – to take action to create a beautiful and meaningful life.

So as we ask for assistance, we then do our best to help move things forward in the direction of our request so that God can work through those potentials set in motion. But, lest we get into our ego about it, there is another important point.

We don't always have the bigger picture. We don't know what ripple effects will happen from our request. Trust, in another sense, is that if I am praying for the Higher Good the outcome may not be what my lower mind would choose. It may not be what I think I want. Just because I want something does not mean it is the best outcome for the entire course of the river of life, which will flow from this point forward. So while we can pray for things and even for specific outcomes, we can ask, "If it is in the highest Good." This expresses some humility and also leaves the door open for something better than we might even imagine to ask for.

Additionally, we never have the right to interfere with another being's free will. While we may love someone and wish with all our heart that they never leave us, that includes the choice a soul makes – at a level beyond the physical – about when it is ready to leave this physical life and move on to its next adventure. I too have experienced loss. While we may grieve the loss of their presence in our life, it is right to give them permission to go when it is their time and to support them in that transition.

Within these sacred boundaries, we have immense power. It is our sacred duty, standing in our power, to take intentional action toward the achievement of the things we wish to see happen. And, in humbleness, to simultaneously acknowledge and work with the higher guidance and Divine order that is at play in all of life.

The Power of Connection

I know talking about this dimension of our existence in the same context as science and medicine is considered taboo, "fantasy" and unscientific to many in our Western medical culture. Spiritual science, or metaphysics, is a real phenomenon as well, whether we choose to accept that or not. It is part of our reality as humans. For us to experience wholeness and balance, which is health itself, healthy spirituality needs to be brought back into the conversation. Otherwise, we are ignoring a huge part of who we are. Without that, we do not understand who we are. If we don't understand who we are, we cannot give attention to all the parts of us that need attention to be healthy here in this physical life, to be successful and to thrive.

We are all connected. We influence each other. We share a very real experience. And our choices affect everyone around us. Whether we are talking about helping your pet heal after a cancer diagnosis, supporting a human loved one through a life crisis, or pursuing your own healing, working to strengthen your connection with the essence of who you are and exploring how you are connected to the universal energies around you is a huge support in allowing you to operate at your full potential. You will be stronger and more balanced. You will be able to weather the storms of life with a steady grip on the sails of your ship to steer yourself through the ever-changing currents of life.

When you are connected, you are able to be present with others in a completely different way. Your inner Sun shines brightly and you are in balance. You, as the sun in your pet's universe, are bright, stable and alive. You become capable of more. Everyone's quality of life improves.

Your healing is not selfish. It is how you serve others from a higher capacity that doesn't burn out your flame at the end of every day. Your healing is, I will be bold enough to say, NOT optional.

Focusing on others first can become an excuse not to heal yourself, so that you can stay small. I'm here to tell you that isn't why you are here. You are here to grow into your potential and to become the magic bullet in your own life so you can help others to the highest of your capacity.

Beyond merely feeling happy and being free of stress and emotional suffering, there is an even deeper potential. It is the essence of the true power and potential you carry within you. We explore this in the next chapter.

CHAPTER 14 CHECK-IN

The power of prayer has been shown to improve recovery and decrease healing time in human patients.

- Practice tuning into your pet's subtler communications. Can you sense what they are telling you? What do they need?
- Pray for your pet and yourself.
- Think about your connection to God.
- Think about how we are all connected, sharing life.

The privilege of a lifetime is to become who you truly are.

– Carl Jung, psychiatrist, psychotherapist, *Memories, Dreams and Reflections*

Chapter 15

The Magic Bullet

We all wish for a magic bullet – that one perfect treatment, supplement or discovery that will make the cancer go away and give us back the life we had before the diagnosis. It's what drives many late-night searches on the internet, the restless questioning of doctors, and the lingering feelings of regret or guilt. *Did I miss something? Could I have found the answer if I had just looked harder?*

This longing is deeply human. When someone we love is suffering, especially our animal companions who rely on us so completely, the instinct to find a cure feels both like a duty and a desperate hope, especially if you are the "Purpose-Driven Pathfinder" type.

No matter what you might have read on the internet, there is no single magical cure that fits every being, every body or every journey. Cancer is not one thing. It is not a singular diagnosis with the same root cause in every patient. If it were that simple, we would have a cure. Cancer is a complex intermingling of dimensions with intricate nuances physically, energetically and spiritually.

Each path through cancer is unique. While medicine, integrative therapies and holistic care can all play vital roles, in the end the greatest source of healing and quality of life for your pet comes from something significantly more personal, more potent and more profound: YOU. You are the one who can weave love and meaning into every moment you and your pet share, through the way you show up, the way you heal, and the way you love.

You may not be able to control how your pet responds to treatment. You can, however, choose how you walk beside them, how you grow through the journey, and how you fill their days with peace, enjoyment and love. That choice, your healing and your presence, is the real magic bullet that gives them the quality of life that you desire for them above everything else, even the cancer cure. Because you want their life to be good. You want them to be free of suffering. You want them to enjoy the time they have as much as possible.

That is important, because the center of your pet's universe is YOU. You are the sun around which their life revolves. And in that, you have power. In many ways, you might feel powerless right now. It is always my advice to focus on what you *do* have power to influence.

Think of how your pet softens when you are calm and centered, or how their eyes light up when you are joyful. The atmosphere shifts and your whole home feels lighter. That is something *you* are doing. You create that! It is a tangible reflection of the power of the human-animal bond and a powerful testament to your ability to improve their quality of life by improving the way you show up in the world.

So when I say you are the magic bullet, I don't mean you carry the burden of finding a cure: I mean that your presence, your choices and your own healing bring the most light, comfort and possibility into your pet's world.

You influence their quality of life in a very meaningful way every day. They feel your energy and calm. You can guide them, and let them guide you in return, into greater peace, acceptance and attention to the precious moments you have together. To me, that is the most beautiful gift – the way we help each other heal and really appreciate the good moments in life, the way we invite each other to create those moments together.

So, how do you become the magic bullet?

You heal and grow. You choose to BECOME the best version of yourself.

You step into your power, not from a place of ego and superiority, but from a place of humility and understanding. You understand that you are the Creator of your life. God works through you. You have power in that connection and that unity. You also have a responsibility for your own life and how you choose to live every day. Additionally, the same is true for everyone else. The question is: How will you use that information?

You have a choice. You can be an agent for Good in your life, if you choose, knowing that you will always be presented with the opportunities to choose differently.

If you desire to bring Good into your life and the world, you must heal all that is antithetical to that within you, so you can be as clear as possible and make the wisest decisions. That process requires forgiveness and grace – forgiveness of others, and most importantly, forgiveness of yourself.

In your healing and growth, you become the lasting legacy of your pet's life and love. Because, in truth, the center of *your* universe is YOU. If your universe is off kilter, that means you have the ability to re-adjust. If this journey with your pet helps you take the steps to move forward in ways you weren't willing to or weren't aware of before, then they have fulfilled their sacred mission with you.

As you move on in your life after their eventual passing – hopefully of old age – the ripple effects of that growth and healing will continue to unfold. Their life will take on a greater meaning through you. In your healing, you can create better relationships with the people in your life. You will be able to operate at a higher capacity and make a more positive difference in the world. And, hopefully, you will carry them in your heart with gratitude for the gift of your time together and all they taught you. Once their time here is done, the echoes of their life will be a healing balm to your grief as you adjust to their absence and create new paths forward to ever and ever greater expressions of Love in the world.

The Last Rite of Passage

Death is a natural part of life. In the Western world, we have become very isolated from the end-of-life experience. It used to be that death was part of society, and in some cultures, death was even honored as a sacred time of transitioning from one type of existence into another. No matter your beliefs, it is helpful to try to come to some peace around the reality that, whether we cure the cancer or not, your pet will eventually leave the world. The important question is: "How well did we live?"

When the time comes to say goodbye, it can be a beautiful practice to make their passing as peaceful and special as possible. You can create a calm environment and even a special little ceremony to honor their life. You can create a beautiful flower bouquet. Light a candle. Play some calming music. Have a special blanket and their favorite toys. Feed them their favorite snacks if they want to eat – maybe something you would never have given them before.

Make their final time here a special goodbye, sending them off to their next adventure. Share some favorite memories. Thank them for all they have brought to your life. Acknowledge what they have taught you. Tell them that you love them and that, although you will miss them, you will be okay. Give them permission to go. They will feel that. As their spirit leaves their body, you might even feel moved to say a special prayer.

Of course you will be sad. You will grieve. Give yourself permission to do this in a healthy way. That sadness is a beautiful testament to the depth of love you allowed yourself to feel. That grief will come in waves. As you get further and further away from the experience, those waves will be less frequent and less intense.

As you experience your emotions, take advantage of the support systems you have around you by talking to someone you trust and who is supportive. Then, actively engage in activities to help you process these emotional experiences. This will help you ultimately accept and integrate the experience of loss. You can then, eventually, come to a place of acceptance and closure, appreciating the gift of the life that was shared with you and the happiness it brought you.

Allowing yourself to express and experience it all can help you move through the grieving process with greater ease and grace. Cry, journal about your feelings and thoughts, create something in memory of your pet, and engage in regular movement or exercise.

Creating new experiences and new routines to fill the hole left by their absence can be a gentle way to help your mind recalibrate to this new reality. You are living and moving forward into a new beginning. It can be especially helpful to create new routines for yourself in spaces where you frequently saw them in life: when you first get home, for example, and are used to being greeted by them. Or when you go to bed and are used to snuggling with them. These are examples of times and spaces where intentionally set new routines can be particularly helpful. Creating these new experiences for yourself will help your brain adjust to the new reality of life without them by your side.

Most importantly, remember that the love you experienced with your pet wasn't *from* them. They just helped you realize the love within your own heart. They helped draw that love to the surface. You can, now, call that love up to guide you in how to be more loving and accepting toward the humans in your life. It is this experience of unconditional love from our pets that ultimately heals us, and that they leave behind with us. It is their gift, their legacy, to humanity.

What You Can Do Now

There are many ways to work with the information I have presented already in this book, starting today. Start where you can, while honoring your current capacities. One small step is better than nothing at all.

If that is all you are ready for right now, it is enough. It is also more than most people will ever do. Be proud of yourself for being strong and taking even one step in a positive direction during this very challenging time. It is through small, consistent steps forward that you create a new and even more amazing life!

Start today incorporating one new routine from each of the Three Cornerstones of Whole-Being Wellness: Physical Body, Soul and Spirit. You will find a practical guide for that in Part V: Daily Alignment Map. This map will provide you with many options to create a daily routine in which you are doing at least one thing to support your Physical Health, Soul Health and Spiritual Health every day.

Chapter 16

Diving Deeper: Bringing Spirituality to Life

As we end this exploration of the pet cancer caregiver journey, let us take a deeper look at how you can make every moment sacred. I think about that as "ritualizing life." How can you make every moment meaningful and bring awareness of the Three Cornerstones of Whole-Being Wellness into everything you do?

One way to bring spirituality into your everyday life is to create small daily practices that connect you with the spiritual dimension. These can be moments of prayer, quiet contemplation, journaling or lighting a candle with intention. Let these practices remind you of the power within you to shift the energy of your day, and in doing so, shift the energy of your pet's life as they share life with you.

A powerful way to take this further is to make everything you do a sacred act, an honoring of life.

- As you prepare their food, bring love into the process. Ritualize the process. Maybe use a special beautiful clean bowl for their meal. Have gratitude for the people involved in making the food. Say a little prayer of healing over it. "May this meal nourish them and support their healing." As you say this prayer, feel the uplifting energy of the Divine moving through you.

- As you give them their medicine or supplements, be present with the process. Ritualize the process. Have gratitude for the access to healing medicines. Imagine your pet healthy and thriving and how the medicines will help them heal.
- As you play with them, appreciate the moment. Life is sacred and beautiful. See if you can imagine the thread of the Divine running through them and you. The connection of Love. Allow yourself to feel happy, to enjoy and to laugh.
- As you snuggle with them, appreciate the healing power of connection. Have gratitude for the time you have. Maybe make that connection time a nightly ritual, where you light a candle and relax and tell them three good things that happened that day.
- Allow this way of living to infuse everything that you do with the people in your life too. What has your pet taught you about the power of relationships and love?

As much as you can, work from a place of love for yourself and others. Love your pet and allow that love you feel to fill you up and ripple out into the rest of your life. Connect with the energy of Love in all you do.

Are You Looking for More?

As you grow through this journey, you may feel called to go deeper into these mysteries and learn ancient, sacred tools that awaken your ability to create peace, clarity and resilience on purpose, not just by accident. There is a way to engage with intentional daily practices that increases the power of what you do, catalyzes your growth, and awakens new potentials within you. Ritual practice in a true spiritual lineage aligned with the Divine powerfully connects to higher spiritual energy and brings that into your life. It makes everything you do matter even more. If one day you desire to explore the deeper spiritual teachings of a true Mystery School, there are keys waiting for you – keys that unlock an even greater experience of your own light and the life you were always meant to live. I can help you begin. If you are ready and seeking more, you are invited to explore this further with me in the book's Afterword.

There, I invite you into the world of Spirit and fields of potential by introducing you to a path of spiritual awakening available to anyone who desires it. This is a path of universal spirituality, and it is for everyone, everywhere: all traditions and religions and beliefs. It is not something of my own invention; it is an ancient hermetic Mystery School lineage. It isn't a religion; it is a path and a way of living that brings spirituality and physicality together. Because it is not religious, there is no dogma. You may, however, recognize spiritual concepts that have become part of various religions. It is a way of more deeply understanding life and the meaning of life. It is a way of living in greater spiritual alignment with who you truly are, with the Divine; it empowers you to reach your human potential.

You, my dear, are extra-ordinary. You might just not know that yet. You might not accept it yet. But with healing, you can. Nothing, however, is required. You are here to explore and to make your own choices. This life is like a "choose your own adventure" book. Are you old enough to remember those? At each fork in the road, you have a choice. Do you go left or do you go right? What flows from your choices leads to any number of new adventures, new challenges and new opportunities. That is the amazing journey we are on called Life. What will you do with yours? Will you get lost in the chaos and swept along in the current? Or will you stand up and forge your path forward?

You can begin to awaken to your higher potential right now, through the choices you make each day and the way you live your life in greater awareness of your power to create change. In this book, I have been walking you through a journey that allows you, if you choose, to start to turn a painful situation into an opportunity for growth. We are transforming a cancer diagnosis into a path to deeper Soul-level healing for both you and your pet. So, in a sense, you are already tasting the essence of it.

You may already recognize times when you've transformed a moment. Each time you chose presence over panic, hope over despair, compassion over anger, you shifted the world around you. You changed your pet's experience simply by the way you showed up. That is the quiet, powerful transformational power of Love in action. That is available to you right now. And it is just the tip of the iceberg.

The healthier, calmer and more resilient you are, the more you create an environment of love, peace and comfort for them. The more you grow through this journey – learning to nurture your own body, soothe your own emotions, deepen your own spirit, and live in alignment with your higher purpose – the more you offer your pet the very best of life during the time you have together. Your healing becomes the alchemy that transforms their life experience too.

If the deeper spiritual aspects of life are inspiring to you or you are looking for something more, what I offer in the Afterword is for you.

Part IV Takeaway

Spiritual Health

Focus on Spiritual Body Health

- Do one thing every day to feed your Spirit.
- Aspire to make every moment sacred.
- Connect with something bigger than yourself every day.
- Remember that there is often more to life than what we see on the surface.
- Try out some new ways to bring meaningful ritual into your days.

Activity Ideas

- Journal a free-flow conversation with God/Universe every day.
- Light a candle and reflect on the Divine in yourself, in your pet and in the world.
- Sit quietly and imagine you are being filled with Light from the top of your head, the light of God or the Divine, and that this nourishes you. Then imagine sending that Light from your heart to your pet.
- Pray for assistance to help you know what to do and how to do it.
- Read a passage from a spiritual text.

- You can do all of these while sitting with your pet, enjoying their company. They feel your energy shift. You might notice they enjoy it and seek you out when you are in these quiet, connected moments.

Esoteric Contemplation Invitation

- Look your pet in the eye and tell them you love them. Really see them.
- Look yourself in the eye, in the mirror, and say "I love you" three times. Really see yourself.

The greatest gift our animal companions often leave us is not merely memories – it is the person we become because we loved them.

Conclusion

I hope what you have read in these pages has inspired you and given you some positive things to focus on in creating new supportive daily routines.

As I said at the beginning, ultimately, simply reading this book itself won't change anything. What you choose to change and DO every day with what you learn creates the momentum to move you forward into a new way of being. This book is a road map, and you don't just read a road map. You use it to chart the path to a destination, and then you physically follow those steps or that path. It's not just in your mind, intention and thoughts. You take action in real life.

Following are two Daily Alignment Maps, which provide Whole-Being Wellness activities from which I encourage you to create a new daily routine that nurtures all Three Cornerstones of Whole-Being Wellness: Body, Soul and Spirit. The first focuses on you. The second focuses on activities you can do with your pet. Choose the activities that resonate most with you. Which ones will work the best for you? The ones you will actually *do* every day.

Start by choosing one from each category – Body, Soul and Spirit – and work those into your daily routine. Stick with it for 30 days to allow yourself time to get into the flow. Create new daily routines that support you and your pet as you navigate this journey. If you are adventurous, choose more than one from each category. Remember, though, consistency in each area is more important than "doing more."

With consistent daily practice, you will make slow, steady progress and notice shifts. Keep a journal of your experiences to track your progress. This helps you recognize the positive changes you make, especially gradual changes you might not notice right away. Months later, when you revisit your journal entries, you may see their powerful impacts.

The choices you make each moment matter. Every day is an opportunity to intentionally impact the direction your life unfolds and to transform the way you show up for yourself and those you love. This is about much more than simply thinking positively. It is about the ways that you, as a spiritual being, actively participate in the trajectory of your life. You have a deep well of strength that you can call forward, at any time, to support you. The practices in this book will help you access that well and support you in creating a Whole-Being Wellness lifestyle, for both you and your pet.

Remember, you are powerful! You are important. You matter, and you can do anything you set your mind to doing. You are also not alone. I am here to help if you are willing to travel. And, if not me, there are people around the globe who have dedicated their lives to helping others. Lean on the resources available to you until you are able to stand strong in your newfound peace and power. Spend time every day nurturing your Body, Soul and Spirit. What you learn about yourself through this journey might surprise you.

Your life is a potent ripple in the fabric of time. What if this journey with your pet brings you into a greater sense of purpose, a greater capacity to live the life you know you were meant to live? That is a legacy of Light worthy of the life you have taken into your care. And your pet will live on through that legacy...You.

DAILY ALIGNMENT MAPS

Whole-Being Wellness

How to use this chart:

Each day, choose **one practice from each area** – Body, Soul and Spirit – to create a balanced self-care practice. By tending to your own Whole-Being Wellness, you not only thrive but also show up more fully for your beloved animal companions.

Body (Physical Wellness)
Eat a nourishing, whole-food meal instead of skipping or grabbing fast food
Take a brisk walk, do yoga or move your body for at least 20 minutes
Drink at least 8 glasses of clean water
Schedule and attend regular health checkups
Practice gentle stretching before bed to release tension
Get 7–8 hours of restorative sleep
Take supplements or herbs that support your health (as guided by a professional)
Limit caffeine, alcohol and screen time
Move your body outdoors – sunlight exposure for vitamin D

Soul (Mind & Emotional Wellness)
Practice 5–10 minutes of meditation or deep breathing
Journal your thoughts, feelings or insights from the day for 5 minutes before bed
Call or meet a supportive friend or loved one
Spend intentional time in nature (walk barefoot, listen to birds, observe trees)
Receive or practice energy healing (Reiki, breathwork, Life Activation, Aura Healing, etc.)
Make a gratitude list of three things you appreciate today
Engage in a creative hobby (painting, music, writing, gardening)
Read an uplifting book or listen to an inspiring podcast
Practice mindful breathing when feeling stressed

Spirit (Deeper Meaning & Connection)
Spend a few minutes in prayer or gratitude for life's blessings, even if they are very small things right now
Contemplate your life purpose and how you're living in alignment with it
Read a passage from a spiritual or inspirational text
Light a candle and reflect on the Divine in yourself and the world
Create a simple daily ritual that honors your Spirit (altar time, morning blessing, evening reflection)
Spend time in silence, cultivating presence and listening inwardly
Stargaze, moon-watch or reflect on your connection to the cosmos
Set an intention for your day and align your actions with it
Visualize yourself surrounded by light and connected to all life

Whole-Being Wellness Activities to Do Together

How to use this chart:

Each day (or week), choose **one practice from each area** – Body, Soul and Spirit – to create a balanced wellness practice that nourishes you and your pet on every level.

Body (Physical Well-Being)
Prepare a fresh, balanced, species-appropriate meal
Take a daily walk or gentle hike together
Engage in playful movement (fetch, tug, agility, hide-and-seek; for cats: chasing a laser light or feather toy)
Provide regular veterinary checkups and preventive care
Practice gentle stretching or yoga with your pet in the room
Offer therapeutic touch or massage to ease tension and improve circulation
Ensure adequate hydration and clean water daily
Provide enrichment toys or puzzles to stimulate physical activity

Soul (Mind & Emotional Well-Being)

Practice mindful petting or grooming, noticing texture, breath and bond

Meditate with your pet nearby; focus on breath and calm presence

Journal about what your pet has taught you about love, patience or resilience

Connect with nature together – sit quietly outdoors, listen to birds, notice surroundings

Try an energy healing practice (Reiki, Life Activation or Aura Balancing) and also schedule one for your pet

Create a "gratitude list" including qualities you appreciate in your pet
Create a "bucket list" for your pet, and each week or month do one thing on the list

Play calming music and relax together in intentional rest

Visualize a sphere of light around you and your pet, filling with calm and safety, and imagine healing for you both

Spirit (Deeper Meaning & Connection)

Spend a few minutes in prayer or gratitude, giving thanks for your pet's presence

Contemplate the deeper purpose of your life and your pet's role as teacher/companion

Read a sacred or inspirational text aloud in your pet's presence

Light a candle or create a simple ritual honoring your pet as a soul companion

Reflect on the human-animal bond as a mirror of the Divine in all life

Hold space for silence together and sense the sacredness in your shared stillness

Set an intention for your day and invite your pet's presence into that prayer

Spend time stargazing or moon-watching with your pet, reflecting on cosmic connection

Ultimately, the purpose of healing is not simply to overcome illness or alleviate suffering – it is to awaken to the fullest expression of what it means to be truly alive. Sometimes the journey we begin for someone we love becomes the journey that transforms us.

Afterword

Invitation to Healing, Greater Connection and Expanded Awareness

Caring for a beloved pet through a cancer diagnosis is one of the most tender and challenging experiences a pet parent can face. It asks more of the heart than we ever expect, and it often brings us into deeper contact with our fears, our hopes and the parts of ourselves we don't always slow down to notice. Healing in this context is not only about medical decisions or symptom management. It is also about supporting YOU: your resilience, your clarity and your ability to stay grounded and connected while navigating uncertainty. When you grow, your pet feels it. When you find steadiness, they rest more easily. When you cultivate peace, you create a healing environment for both of you.

For some, this journey opens a door for them to want to explore additional support and deeper healing. It might awaken a Soul-deep desire to step into greater self-mastery or awakening. For some who are already spiritually oriented, the cancer journey may connect you with avenues of growth you were not aware were available before and awaken a new excitement for learning and spiritual mastery.

If you are one of the people who are interested in more, there is a path to growth, healing and expanded consciousness that works on a quantum level, expanding your consciousness. This path is available to all, including you. It works at the level of your spiritual blueprint, awakening dormant potential waiting to propel you into an elevated expression of your life and personal mission. It is a path that can clear subconscious programs that keep you in repeating patterns. It can help you break through limitations into greater levels of peace, freedom and mastery in your life.

The only way I know of and that I can recommend in integrity is the one I have personally experienced to be in alignment with the Light and also effective at this level. Because it works beyond the thoughts and emotions, this way of accessing healing often does not make sense to the mind. It is not logical. It is spiritual. It speaks to the Soul.

For brave and courageous Souls seeking for more, I invite you to step onto a path of healing I have learned as an initiate in one of the few remaining true Mystery Schools on the planet. These are not *my* ideas, methods or techniques; they are modalities preserved through antiquity in an ancient lineage of Light. It is a true Path of Empowerment in which there is no limit to your continued growth other than what you choose for yourself. If you are ready to put in the work to break through the ways you are holding yourself back and expand your understanding of yourself, God and the universe, then this is a great path for you. Ultimately, it is a path for those who want to make the world a better place and who understand that peace starts within. Only when we learn to live from that place of inner peace ourselves can we be a force for Peace and Hope in the world.

It is not an "easy" path. True healing doesn't always feel "good" or "comfortable." It can be challenging as you are going through it. Why? Because by getting to the root of the things that keep you stuck, you may need to question your beliefs – to challenge them in order to discover if they are keeping you stuck in old patterns. It can require you to face your fears and your shadows, even uncomfortable truths about your current state. It asks you to bring light into the shadowy places inside you so you can clear the cobwebs and repair areas that are keeping you from moving forward. There is a strength required to heal, but you have that strength inside you. We all do. And it is the most rewarding work you can do.

I will repeat what I said in Chapter 14:

God/Universe/Spirit is inside of you; God is a part of who you are. As you connect with that part of yourself, under your own power, using tools that empower you to clear up that connection without compromising your sovereignty, authority, autonomy and your inner connection to the Source of All Things, you heal at a core level. You feel connected not just in moments, but throughout your entire day. You are clear. You can then move in your life in a completely different way.

Invitation to Work with Me

If you are ready for this Great Work and would like to connect with me to take your first steps, you can visit my website. The first step for most people is a Life Activation. This is an energy activation session that, when provided by a qualified practitioner, re-ignites your Divine blueprint and connects you with more clarity to your Divine essence, the part of you that remembers God in the bigger sense of the word. It awakens the part of you that remembers who you are and your life purpose. This is a gentle but powerful healing. Many will just receive this activation and go on with their life, allowing greater clarity to gradually unfold through the choices they make.

Others, like me, will choose to continue on a path of progression into greater spiritual awakening with the goal of healing and becoming a more balanced and aligned Light Leader in the world.

In the ancient Mystery School tradition, healings and classes are done in person. We honor the way these sacred teachings have been handed down through the centuries, in an oral tradition and direct transmission. You can read information, of course: There is no shortage of information available these days, and if you want to do it on your own, you are welcome to make that choice. Books are helpful in that regard. You can satisfy your mental curiosity and consider new information you might not have considered before. When you are ready to move beyond information into embodiment, living in a way that you have not yet been able to reach on your own, that requires an in-person experience, and the willingness to be mentored.

Use discernment when taking a teacher, as not everyone is worthy of your trust and attention. Investigate their credentials. Are they embodying and living something you desire to achieve for yourself? Are they living in integrity? Do they hold themselves accountable to anyone else? Are they still actively learning and growing themselves? Every good teacher is also a student, always. Search your heart; only you will know the path that is right for you. A Good path teaches you how to think for yourself, to question, and to arrive at your own conclusions based on the new information you are given. It also teaches you how to live in alignment with the Light in this world of polarities, a complex and sometimes confusing interaction of Light and Dark. This is the path of the true Mystery School tradition: the path to "Know Thyself."

I am here to help you, if and when you are ready. I offer healings, workshops and spiritual training intensives regularly throughout the year. If you would like to find someone closer to you who is properly trained and has maintained their certification, I can help you with that as well.

Work With Me

Acknowledgments

A deep thank you to my many teachers and mentors, most notably:

Dr. Steve Marsden, healer extraordinaire, whose brilliant mind, patience and generous spirit taught me the art of veterinary Chinese herbal medicine. He has been an amazing mentor and for this I am deeply grateful. Through A Time to Heal advanced herbal courses and the College of Integrative Veterinary Therapies, as well as countless hours of his personal time, he has supported me in developing a degree of expertise in Chinese herbal medicine that has allowed me to help thousands of pets and dedicated pet parents, opening a door of healing that many would not have known existed for veterinary patients.

My mentors and teachers: Gudni Gudnason, founder of the Modern Mystery School, Sovereign Ipsissimus Dave Lanyon, and Sovereign Ipsissimus Hideto Nakagokme, lineage holders in the Mystery School tradition of King Salomon, one of the few true Mystery Schools that still exists on the planet. Under their mentorship and guidance, I have had the privilege of studying the deeper esoteric healing methods and living the initiatory path kept pure and protected through the lineage. I have a huge amount of respect and gratitude for their integrity and the rare example of stability, consistency and kindness that they embody. It is from the body of wisdom preserved and made available to the public through their efforts that I have acquired the skill and capacity to provide deeper levels of support for my clients, who are also looking for the help and deep healing I needed to find the inner peace I was seeking.

Finally, I thank Life's greatest teacher: the challenges I have faced and grown beyond that have made me the person I am today. They provided the fertile ground for me to learn how to live life better, realize my strengths, transform my weaknesses, achieve more happiness and joy in my life, and continue to grow into better and better versions of myself every day.

Appendix

The Life Activation

Whether it's a difficult diagnosis, the weight of making the "right" decisions for your pet, or simply the emotional toll of walking this cancer journey, you don't have to navigate it alone. There is a way to reconnect with your clarity, peace and inner strength in a way that works on your foundation, underneath your busy thoughts and turbulent emotions. This healing session is one of the most powerful tools I've experienced for helping people move out of fear and overwhelm and into greater calm, inner peace and clarity.

Life Activation has helped clients I have worked with to:

- Make more aligned and confident decisions
- Feel more peaceful, even in the face of uncertainty
- Reconnect with the inner guidance in a gentle way
- Clear mental and emotional fog
- Tap into their deeper sense of purpose and power

Life Activation is an in-person session that opens the door to a whole new level of awareness and healing. The results are personal. While many clients share they experience immediate shifts like feeling lighter and calmer, the results tend to unfold gradually over time. Clients often tell me things just start to "click" afterward. That they feel like a "weight has been lifted" and are better able to make decisions. Often they will say they feel "like themselves again." You don't need to have it all figured out; you just need to take the next step.

This session may support you in staying present and help you connect with a sense of inner peace so you can be more present for your pet, have more clarity as you navigate difficult decisions, and hold space for them in a different way. But you don't have to be supporting a pet through cancer to benefit from this session. This session may also be powerful for anyone looking to connect with more clarity around their life direction and personal growth.

To learn more about my other healing services, spiritual training, workshops, retreats and meditation events, visit www.drerinbannink.com.

Endnotes

1 "About the Comparative Oncology Program," Center for Cancer Research, National Cancer Institute, https://ccr.cancer.gov/comparative-oncology-program/about.

2 Claudia M. Witt et al., "A Comprehensive Definition for Integrative Oncology," JNCI Monographs 2017, no. 52 (November 2017), https://doi.org/10.1093/jncimonographs/lgx012.

3 C. M. Jantien Vrijmoet-Wiersma et al., "Assessment of Parental Psychological Stress in Pediatric Cancer: A Review," Journal of Pediatric Psychology 33, no. 7 (August 2008): 694–706, https://doi.org/10.1093/jpepsy/jsn007.

4 Anna-Lena Norberg and Krister K. Boman, "Parent Distress in Childhood Cancer: A Comparative Evaluation of Posttraumatic Stress Symptoms, Depression and Anxiety," Acta Oncologica 47, no. 2 (2008): 267–74, https://doi.org/10.1080/02841860701558714.

5 B. A. Sisk, S. Weng, and J. W. Mack, "Persistently Low Peace of Mind in Parents of Cancer Patients: A Five-Year Follow-up Study," Pediatric Blood & Cancer 66, no. 5 (May 2019): e27609, https://doi.org/10.1002/pbc.27609.

6 Luz Endo-Munoz et al., "Auranofin Improves Overall Survival When Combined with Standard of Care in a Pilot Study Involving Dogs with Osteosarcoma," Veterinary and Comparative Oncology 18, no. 2 (June 2020): 206–13.

7 Marcio C. Machado et al., "The Effect of Naltrexone as a Carboplatin Chemotherapy-Associated Drug on the Immune Response, Quality of Life and Survival of Dogs with Mammary Carcinoma," PLoS One 13, no. 10 (October 2018): e0204830.

8 X. W. Zhang et al., "Acupuncture for Cancer-Related Conditions: An Overview of Systematic Reviews," Phytomedicine 106 (November 2022): 154430.

9 M. Faria et al., "Efficacy of Acupuncture on Cancer Pain: A Systematic Review and Meta-Analysis," Journal of Integrative Medicine 22, no. 3 (May 2024): 235–44.

10 T. R. de Sousa et al., "Acupuncture Techniques and Acupoints Used in Individuals under Chemotherapy or Radiotherapy Treatment of Cancer: A Systematic Review," Journal of Clinical Nursing 32, no. 19-20 (October 2023): 6917–33.

11 Y. J. Zhu et al., "Acupuncture for Quality of Life in Gastric Cancer Patients Undergoing Adjuvant Chemotherapy," Journal of Pain and Symptom Management 63, no. 2 (February 2022): 210–20.

12 J. Nian et al., "Efficacy and Safety of Acupuncture for Chemotherapy-Induced Leukopenia: A Systematic Review and Meta-Analysis," Medicine 101, no. 42 (October 21, 2022): e30995.

13 A. Castelló et al., "High Adherence to Western Dietary Pattern Increases Breast Cancer Risk (An EPIC-Spain Study)," Maturitas 179 (January 2024): 107868.

14 T. Lan et al., "Plant-Based, Fast-Food, Western-Contemporary, and Animal-Based Dietary Patterns and Risk of Premature Aging in Adult Survivors of Childhood Cancer: A Cross-Sectional Study," BMC Medicine 23, no. 1 (February 25, 2025): 120.

15 A. Campanella et al., "Ultra-Processed Food Consumption as a Risk Factor for Gastrointestinal Cancer and Other Causes of Mortality in Southern Italy: A Competing Risk Approach," Nutrients 16, no. 13 (June 23, 2024): 1994.

16 M. Mahmoodi et al., "The Association between Healthy and Unhealthy Dietary Indices with Prostate Cancer Risk: A Case-Control Study," Journal of Health, Population and Nutrition 43, no. 1 (June 20, 2024): 90.

17 L. Zhao et al., "Ultra-Processed Products and Risk of Liver Cancer: A Prospective Cohort Study," Clinical Nutrition 43, no. 10 (October 2024): 2298–304.

18 J. Barbaresko et al., "Ultra-Processed Food Consumption and Human Health: An Umbrella Review of Systematic Reviews with Meta-Analyses," Critical Reviews in Food Science and Nutrition 65, no. 11 (2025): 1999–2007.

19 I. M. Isaksen and S. N. Dankel, "Ultra-Processed Food Consumption and Cancer Risk: A Systematic Review and Meta-Analysis," Clinical Nutrition 42, no. 6 (June 2023): 919–28.

20 T. Fiolet et al., "Consumption of Ultra-Processed Foods and Cancer Risk: Results from NutriNet-Santé Prospective Cohort," BMJ 360 (February 14, 2018): k322.

21 D. Hang et al., "Ultra-Processed Food Consumption and Risk of Colorectal Cancer Precursors: Results from 3 Prospective Cohorts," Journal of the National Cancer Institute 115, no. 2 (February 8, 2023): 155–64.

22 A. Al Nahas et al., "Associations between Degree of Food Processing and Colorectal Cancer Risk in a Large-Scale European Cohort," International Journal of Cancer 157, no. 2 (July 15, 2025): 260–76.

23 M. Mahmoudi-Zadeh et al., "The Association between Ultra-Processed Foods Intake and the Odds of Prostate Cancer: A Case-Control Study," Journal of Health, Population and Nutrition 44, no. 1 (April 1, 2025): 97.

24 M. Nouri et al., "Association between Processed and Ultra-Processed Food Intake and the Risk of Breast Cancer: A Case-Control Study," BMC Cancer 24, no. 1 (October 7, 2024): 1234.

25 M. Song and E. Giovannucci, "Preventable Incidence and Mortality of Carcinoma Associated with Lifestyle Factors among White Adults in the United States," JAMA Oncology 2, no. 9 (2016): 1154–61.

26 M. Long et al., "Plasma Metabolomic Signature of a Proinflammatory Diet in Relation to Breast Cancer Risk: A Prospective Cohort Study," American Journal of Clinical Nutrition 121, no. 3 (March 2025): 548–57.

27 P. Wang et al., "Optimal Dietary Patterns for Prevention of Chronic Disease," Nature Medicine 29, no. 3 (March 2023): 719–28.

28 M. Tajan and K. H. Vousden, "Dietary Approaches to Cancer Therapy," Cancer Cell 37, no. 6 (June 2020): 767–85.

29 V. D. Longo and R. M. Anderson, "Nutrition, Longevity and Disease: From Molecular Mechanisms to Interventions," Cell 185, no. 9 (2022): 1455–70.

30 S. R. Taylor et al., "Developing Dietary Interventions as Therapy for Cancer," Nature Reviews Cancer 22, no. 8 (August 2022): 452–66.

31 J. W. Locasale et al., "Diet and Cancer Metabolism," Cold Spring Harbor Perspectives in Medicine 14, no. 12 (December 2, 2024): a041549.

32 H. J. Thompson, Z. Zhu, and W. Jiang, "Dietary Energy Restriction in Breast Cancer Prevention," Journal of Mammary Gland Biology and Neoplasia 8, no. 1 (January 2003): 133–42.

33 R. J. Colman, R. M. Anderson, S. C. Johnson, et al., "Caloric Restriction Delays Disease Onset and Mortality in Rhesus Monkeys," Science 325, no. 5937 (July 2009): 201–204.

34 E. M. Mercken et al., "Of Mice and Men: The Benefits of Caloric Restriction, Exercise, and Mimetics," Ageing Research Reviews 11, no. 3 (July 2012): 390–98.

35 C. Lee et al., "Fasting Cycles Retard Growth of Tumors and Sensitize a Range of Cancer Cell Types to Chemotherapy," Science Translational Medicine 4, no. 124 (March 7, 2012): 124ra27.

36 I. Caffa et al., "Fasting-Mimicking Diet and Hormone Therapy Induce Breast Cancer Regression," Nature 583, no. 7817 (July 23, 2020): 620–24.

37 M. Di Tano et al., "Synergistic Effect of Fasting-Mimicking Diet and Vitamin C Against KRAS Mutated Cancers," Nature Communications 11, no. 1 (May 11, 2020): 2332.

38 A. Golonko et al., "Dietary Factors and Their Influence on Immunotherapy Strategies in Oncology: A Comprehensive Review," Cell Death & Disease 15, no. 4 (April 9, 2024): 254.

39 J. Zhao et al., "Detection of Glyphosate Residues in Companion Animal Feeds," Environmental Pollution 243, pt. B (December 2018): 1113–18.

40 D. Hunter et al., "Evaluation of the Micronutrient Composition of Plant Foods Produced by Organic and Conventional Agricultural Methods," Critical Reviews in Food Science and Nutrition 51, no. 6 (July 2011): 571–82.

41 M. Rani and S. Kapoor, "Diverse Farming Systems and Their Impact on Macro and Microelement Content of Vegetables & Crops," Recent Advances in Food, Nutrition & Agriculture 15, no. 3 (2024): 204–14.

42 K. Hiney et al., "Clinical Health Markers in Dogs Fed Raw Meat-Based or Commercial Extruded Kibble Diets," Journal of Animal Science 99, no. 6 (June 1, 2021): skab133.

43 S. Cannas et al., "Stress and Cancer in Dogs: Comparison between a Population of Dogs with Cancer and a Population of Healthy Dogs," Macedonian Veterinary Review 39, no. 2 (2016): 201–8.

44 J. H. de Groot et al., "A Sniff of Happiness," Psychological Science 26, no. 6 (2015): 684–700.

45 G. R. Semin et al., "Inter- and Intra-species Communication of Emotion: Chemosignals as the Neglected Medium," Animals 9, no. 11 (2019): 887.

46 B. D'Aniello et al., "Interspecies Transmission of Emotional Information via Chemosignals: From Humans to Dogs (Canis lupus familiaris)," Animal Cognition 21, no. 1 (2018): 67–78.

47 B. D'Aniello et al., "Sex Differences in the Behavioral Responses of Dogs Exposed to Human Chemosignals of Fear and Happiness," Animal Cognition 24, no. 2 (2021): 299–309.

48 C. S. Ozturk and E. Katikol, "Effect of mHealth-based Relaxation Program on Stress Coping and Anxiety Levels in Mothers of Children with Cancer: A Randomized Controlled Study," Patient Education and Counseling 123 (June 2024): 108247.

49 M. Antonelli, G. Barbieri, and D. Donelli, "Effects of Forest Bathing (Shinrin-yoku) on Levels of Cortisol as a Stress Biomarker: A Systematic Review and Meta-analysis," International Journal of Biometeorology 63, no. 8 (2019): 1117–34.

50 L. Queirolo et al., "Effects of Forest Bathing (Shinrin-yoku) in Stressed People," Frontiers in Psychology 15 (2024): 1458418, https://doi.org/10.3389/fpsyg.2024.1458418.

51 J. Li et al., "Prevalence and Influencing Factors of the Dyadic Psychological Stress among Patients with Lung Cancer and Their Family Caregivers: A Cross-sectional Study," BMC Nursing 24, no. 1 (2025): 13, https://doi.org/10.1186/s12912-024-02554-7.

52 V. Yepez et al., "AutoFOCUS: A Mindfulness-Based Intervention for Caregivers of Autologous Hematopoietic Stem Cell Transplant Recipients," Palliative and Supportive Care 23 (2025): e147, https://doi.org/10.1017/S147895152400115X.

53 P. J. Slater, R. M. Edwards, and A. A. Badat, "Evaluation of a Staff Well-Being Program in a Pediatric Oncology, Hematology, and Palliative Care Services Group," Journal of Healthcare Leadership 10 (2018): 67–85.

54 J. N. Donald, B. K. Sahdra, B. Van Zanden, et al., "Does Your Mindfulness Benefit Others? A Systematic Review and Meta-Analysis of the Link Between Mindfulness and Prosocial Behaviour," British Journal of Psychology 110, no. 1 (2019): 101–125.

55 M. Lamothe, É. Rondeau, C. Malboeuf-Hurtubise, et al., "Outcomes of MBSR or MBSR-Based Interventions in Health Care Providers: A Systematic Review with a Focus on Empathy and Emotional Competencies," Complementary Therapies in Medicine 24 (2016): 19–28.

56 C. E. Mosher, K. A. Beck-Coon, et al., "Mindfulness to Enhance Quality of Life and Support Advance Care Planning: A Pilot Randomized Controlled Trial for Adults with Advanced Cancer and Their Family Caregivers," BMC Palliative Care 23, no. 1 (2024): 232.

57 E. A. Hoge, E. Bui, M. Mete, et al., "Mindfulness-Based Stress Reduction vs Escitalopram for the Treatment of Adults With Anxiety Disorders: A Randomized Clinical Trial," JAMA Psychiatry 80, no. 1 (2023): 13–21.

58 R. Jerath, M. W. Crawford, V. A. Barnes, and K. Harden, "Self-Regulation of Breathing as a Primary Treatment for Anxiety," Applied Psychophysiology and Biofeedback 40, no. 2 (2015): 107–115.

59 B. G. Kalyani, G. Venkatasubramanian, R. Arasappa, et al., "Neurohemodynamic Correlates of 'OM' Chanting: A Pilot Functional Magnetic Resonance Imaging Study," International Journal of Yoga 4, no. 1 (2011): 3–6.

60 A. Bowman, F. Dowell, and N. Evans, "The Effect of Different Genres of Music on the Stress Levels of Kennelled Dogs," Physiology & Behavior 171 (2017): 207–215.

61 S. Telke, B. Leininger, L. Hanson, et al., "A Randomized Trial of 21 Days of Loving Kindness Meditation for Stress Reduction and Emotional Well-being Within an Online Health Community for Patients, Family, and Friends Experiencing a Cancer Health Journey," Journal of Integrative and Complementary Medicine 28, no. 2 (2022): 158–167.

62 Y. Zhang, R. Tang, D. Wang, et al., "Family-Centered Online Positive Psychological Intervention for Breast Cancer Patients and Family Caregivers: A Single-Arm Pre-Post Study of Feasibility and Preliminary Effects," BMC Psychology 13, no. 1 (2025): 310.

63 M. L. Sprengel, L. Teo, S. Allen, et al., "Biofield Therapies Clinical Research Landscape: A Scoping Review and Interactive Evidence Map," Journal of Integrative and Complementary Medicine 31, no. 5 (May 2025): 406–430.

64 B. S. Barati, et al., "Effectiveness of Photobiomodulation (Low-Level Laser Therapy) on Treatment of Oral Mucositis (OM) Induced by Chemoradiotherapy in Head and Neck Cancer Patients," Journal of Photochemistry and Photobiology B: Biology 264 (March 2025): 113115. W.

65 W. Dai et al., "The Beneficial Effects of High-Intensity Laser Therapy on a Perineal Wound in a Patient with Rectal Cancer: A Case Report," Journal of Wound Care 34, no. Sup4 (April 2025): S22–S24.

66 F. Cornud et al., "Laser-Focused Ablative Therapy for Prostate Cancer and Benign Prostatic Hyperplasia: A Review of Current Applications and Future Directions," Diagnostic and Interventional Imaging, April 16, 2025, S2211-5684(25)00072-5.

67 T. Almeida et al., "Laser Interstitial Thermal Therapy for Recurrent Brain Metastases Following Stereotactic Radiosurgery: A Systematic Review," Expert Review of Neurotherapeutics 25, no. 4 (April 2025): 465–475.

68 U. Özcan Yüce and S. Taşcı, "Effect of Reiki on the Stress Level of Caregivers of Patients with Cancer: Qualitative and Single-Blind Randomized Controlled Trial," Complementary Therapies in Medicine 58 (May 2021): 102708.

69 S. Oz Kahveci, E. Engin, and E. Goker, "The Effect of Reiki Applied to Cancer Patients on Pain, Anxiety, and Stress Levels: A Randomized Controlled Study," Seminars in Oncology Nursing 41, no. 2 (April 2025): 151807.

70 H. Utli, M. Dinç, and M. D. A. Utli, "The Effect of Acupressure or Reiki Interventions on the Levels of Pain and Fatigue of Cancer Patients Receiving Palliative Care: A Randomized Controlled Study," Explore 19, no. 1 (January–February 2023): 91–99.

71 K. Liu et al., "Effects of Reiki Therapy on Quality of Life: A Meta-Analysis of Randomized Controlled Trials," Systematic Reviews 14, no. 1 (March 27, 2025): 72.

72 M. Y. Bayülgen, "The Effect of Reiki on Fatigue Symptoms of Cancer Patients: A Systematic Review," Holistic Nursing Practice, July 23, 2024.

73 K. L. Tsang, L. E. Carlson, and K. Olson, "Pilot Crossover Trial of Reiki Versus Rest for Treating Cancer-Related Fatigue," Integrative Cancer Therapies 6, no. 1 (March 2007): 25–35.

74 G. Gronowicz, E. R. Secor Jr., J. R. Flynn, and L. T. Kuhn, "Human Biofield Therapy Does Not Affect Tumor Size but Modulates Immune Responses in a Mouse Model for Breast Cancer," Journal of Integrative Medicine 14, no. 5 (September 2016): 389–399.

75 P. Yang et al., "Human Biofield Therapy Modulates Tumor Microenvironment and Cancer Stemness in Mouse Lung Carcinoma," Integrative Cancer Therapies 19 (January–December 2020): 1534735420940398.

76 Maciocia, Giovanni. The Practice of Chinese Medicine: The Treatment of Diseases with Acupuncture and Chinese Herbs. 2nd ed., Elsevier, 2003.

77 T. A. Balboni, T. J. VanderWeele, S. D. Doan-Soares, et al., "Spirituality in Serious Illness and Health," JAMA 328, no. 2 (July 12, 2022): 184–97.

78 I. S. La, M. Johantgen, C. L. Storr, et al., "Spirituality Moderates the Relationship between Cancer Caregiver Burden and Depression," Palliative & Supportive Care 22, no. 3 (June 2024): 470–81.

79 T. A. Balboni, "Spirituality in Advanced Cancer: Implications for Care in Oncologic Emergencies," Annals of Palliative Medicine 13, no. 3 (May 2024): 568–74.

80 A. K. Superdock, A. S. Porter, W. Spears, et al., "Spiritual Communication Between Pediatric Oncologists, Caregivers, and Patients With Brain Tumors," Pediatric Blood & Cancer 72, no. 7 (July 2025): e31721.

81 N. H. Mehta, M. Prajapati, R. Aeleti, et al., "The Power of a Belief System: A Systematic Qualitative Synthesis of Spiritual Care for Patients with Brain Tumors," Journal of Clinical Medicine 13, no. 16 (August 18, 2024): 4871.

82 M. McDarby, M. Miller, W. E. Rosa, et al., "Multidisciplinary Oncology Clinicians' Experiences Delivering Spiritual Care to Patients with Cancer and Their Care Partners," Supportive Care in Cancer 32, no. 9 (August 13, 2024): 586.

83 M. J. Sheridan, "Predicting the Use of Spiritually-Derived Interventions in Social Work Practice: A Survey of Practitioners," Journal of Religion & Spirituality in Social Work: Social Thought 23, no. 1 (2004): 5–25.

84 R. Spatuzzi, M. V. Giulietti, M. Ricciuti, et al., "Exploring the Associations Between Spiritual Well-Being, Burden, and Quality of Life in Family Caregivers of Cancer Patients," Palliative and Supportive Care 17, no. 3 (2019): 294–99.

85 N. Czyżowska, M. Raszka, A. Kalus, and D. Czyżowska, "Posttraumatic Growth and Spirituality in Mothers of Children with Pediatric Cancer," International Journal of Environmental Research and Public Health 18, no. 6 (March 12, 2021): 2890.

86 P. M. Vigna, I. de Castro, and R. L. Fumis, "Spirituality Alleviates the Burden on Family Members Caring for Patients Receiving Palliative Care Exclusively," BMC Palliative Care 19, no. 1 (June 3, 2020): 77.

87 D. K. Bitēna, I. Salmane-Kuļikovska, J. Duhovska, et al., "Spirituality as a Means of Adaptation to Life and Illness for Oncology Patients: A Scoping Review of Quantitative Studies between 2019 and 2025," Journal of Religion and Health 65, no. 1 (February 2026): 408–32.

88 M. Ahmadi, K. Zaree, A. Kazemnejad Leily, and A. S. Sadat Hoseini, "Efficacy of a Written Prayer Technique on the Anxiety of Mothers of Children with Cancer," Palliative & Supportive Care 17, no. 1 (February 2019): 54–59.

About the Author

Dr. Erin Bannink has spent more than two decades sitting in exam rooms with pet parents on some of the hardest days of their lives. As a board-certified veterinary oncologist, she has guided families through the uncertainties and fears that accompany a cancer diagnosis – helping them navigate complex medical decisions while acknowledging the deep emotional bond and love they share with their animals.

Over time, she noticed something that medicine alone could not fully explain. Some patients and their people seemed to find a different kind of peace and surprising levels of healing. Others struggled not just with the diagnosis, but with the weight of fear, overwhelm and disconnection. It became clear there was an aspect to healing that was not just physical. It was emotional. It was spiritual. It was relational.

This realization set Dr. Bannink on a path of exploration beyond conventional medicine. Already grounded in science through her training at Hope College and Michigan State University's College of Veterinary Medicine, she expanded her approach to include acupuncture and Chinese herbal medicine, eventually earning advanced certification and a Graduate Diploma in Veterinary Chinese Herbal Medicine through the College of Integrative Veterinary Therapies. Today, she practices Integrative Oncology at Oakland Veterinary Referral Services in Michigan, blending modern cancer therapies with time-honored healing traditions and lecturing internationally on this integrative approach.

Driven by a desire to understand the deeper forces shaping human and animal experience, she also immersed herself in spiritual study. From early roots in the Christian tradition and Native American shamanic teachings, to years of study in Tibetan Mahayana Buddhism, yogic philosophy and meditation, she followed a path many seekers know well – gathering wisdom, yet still sensing that something essential was missing.

That search ultimately led her to the Western Mystery School tradition – an ancient lineage of spiritual training designed not just to inspire, but to transform and uplift humanity. Today, Dr. Bannink is a Senior Spiritual Guide, healer and metaphysical teacher, in the Hermetic lineage of King Salomon, trained and certified through the Modern Mystery School International. Through this initiatory path, she works with time-tested spiritual technologies passed down for over 3,000 years – tools that activate dormant aspects of the human blueprint and support true self-mastery, clarity and alignment with one's life purpose.

What makes her work unique is her ability to anchor this ancient wisdom into modern life and bridge two worlds that are often kept separate: science and spirit. As an accomplished veterinary specialist, she understands the rigor of evidence-based medicine, the demands of high-performance careers, and the emotional toll of caring deeply in the face of uncertainty. As a spiritual guide, she understands that lasting transformation requires more than knowledge – it requires integration, embodiment and connection to something greater.

Her journey through a high-achieving medical career revealed a reality she now shares openly: External success alone does not create fulfillment. Without alignment, even the most accomplished lives can feel disconnected, heavy or incomplete. True healing – and true purpose – emerge when we begin to bring all parts of ourselves into coherence.

This understanding was shaped not only by her personal path, but by years of witnessing the quiet emotional and spiritual challenges faced by others – pet parents carrying the weight of difficult decisions, veterinary colleagues facing burnout and emotional exhaustion, and high-performing individuals searching for meaning beyond worldly achievement. Through these experiences, Dr. Bannink came to see that healing and fulfillment is not something we acquire from the outside. It is something we cultivate from within.

She is the founder of Divine PowerHouse Center for Healing and Enlightenment, where she offers healing sessions, initiation, classes and workshops designed to support individuals on a path of deep, lasting transformation. Her work is especially resonant for those who feel called to something greater – high-performing individuals and emerging leaders who are ready to move beyond surface-level growth into a life of true inner mastery characterized by clarity, higher purpose and meaningful service.

Her life's work is guided by the understanding that even in our most challenging moments there exists an innate capacity for growth when we learn to honor the interconnected nature of Body, Soul and Spirit – and that within each individual lies the capacity to become a conscious creator of their life and positively impact the world.

www.ingramcontent.com/pod-product-compliance
Lightning Source LLC
LaVergne TN
LVHW050928210926
848482LV00013B/566